The New Rulebook

Notes from a psychologist to help redefine the way you live

Dr Chris Cheers

Harper *by* Design

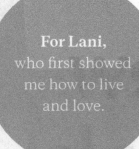

For Lani,
who first showed
me how to live
and love.

I would like to acknowledge that this book was written on the unceded lands of the Wurundjeri People of the Kulin Nation. I pay my respect to Elders past and present. I extend that respect to any Aboriginal and Torres Strait Islander person who is reading this today.

Always was, always will be Aboriginal land.

'If uncertainty is unacceptable to you, it turns into fear. If it is perfectly acceptable, it turns into increased aliveness, alertness, and creativity.'[1]

– Eckhart Tolle

Foreword

We do so much to control the uncertainty of life.

We create rules to live by in the hope that, if we follow them, life will be okay. We choose a career ladder to climb, with the promise that we will find success at the top. We play by all the rules of the game of love, as then we will never be alone. We exercise, eat right, get the grades, do what's expected, and please other people. All for the promise that if we do this, we will be happy.

And when that doesn't work, people come and see me.

As a psychologist, I have sat with many people trying to find relief from the uncertainty of life - people trying to end a relationship, to make a choice, or to have a difficult conversation. And more recently, I have sat with people as they try to deal with the sense of uncertainty brought on by a global pandemic, climate change, and war. People come to me with the hope that there is something I can say that will bring the relief of certainty.

But certainty is not the only way out of the struggle. We can also let go.

We can surrender to the uncertainty. We can accept that much of life is beyond our control; accept that we are never on solid ground; that we can never know the future.

This is how we can view life: not as a series of expectations we must meet, or goals we might fall short of, but as a space of infinite uncertainty. I get it – that sounds terrifying. Why on earth would we ever want to view life like that?

Because that's the reality. And often when we surrender to the reality, we relieve ourselves of the effort it takes to deny it. Accepting things as they are is the starting point for change.

This book is a guide to embracing that uncertainty.

When we embrace uncertainty we are no longer bound to the rules and social structures that we follow to create a certain but artificial reality. We can dismantle the ways we think about wellbeing that are no longer working for us and start to live in a way guided by our needs, our emotions and what is meaningful to us.

This book asks more questions than it answers, because change in your life should start with you. I hope these questions encourage deep thought and self-determined action. I also hope they spark conversations and bring people together. They invite vulnerability, which not only helps us understand ourselves, but also brings us closer to each other.

For many, this time in history is one of great challenge, change and upheaval. Yet if how we were living wasn't working for us, a moment of reckoning is not entirely a bad thing. We have been given space to think about what is meaningful to us and to reflect on how that compares to the rules we have been living by. We are being asked to go back to normal. But what if we want something better?

During times of crisis, I am reminded that I was once taught the term 'crisis' is derived from the Greek 'krisis' meaning 'to sift, decide and discern'.

So, if you are feeling a sense of upheaval in your life right now, consider that in that pain you may also be offered a space to make important choices. To sift and decide what a meaningful life looks like for you.

I want this book to be a guide for your process of reorientation. A guide to help you to re-examine the ways you think about wellness and wellbeing that are not working for you anymore. And to help you live a better life, driven by your own needs.

As a queer man and psychologist who has spent the last decade working with the LGBTIQA+ community, I know that far too often mental health care is presented in a way that is neither accessible nor inclusive. That's why I have written this book – one that people of all genders and sexualities can feel understood and accepted by.

The rulebook for life has been thrown out the window over the past few years. Rather than picking it back up, let's write a new one together.

'And the point is, to live everything. Live the questions now. Perhaps you will then gradually, without noticing it, live along some distant day into the answer.'[2]

– Rainer Maria Rilke

Before we begin

Each section of this book aims to challenge a current way of thinking (old rule) and propose a reframe (new rule). At the end of each section, I offer practical strategies to put these new rules into action.

When you have the capacity to give some of the strategies a go, try to keep focused on the knowledge that changing behaviour is hard and takes time. However, the more compassion you can show yourself as you make change in your life, the more likely change will happen.

I want to acknowledge that the ideas and strategies presented within these pages are informed by my experiences as a white, cisgendered, able-bodied queer man, who has been educated largely through a Western understanding of psychology. While I notice and challenge these biases, I cannot entirely remove myself from them. So as you read through these ideas, keep in mind they are based on that life experience, education, or on the evidence I provide in the endnotes. Take what is helpful and leave behind what is not.

I also appreciate that some of these strategies may not be possible for you because of your specific circumstance and current mental health. If you are currently experiencing significant mental health difficulties, you may have limited capacity to engage with some of the strategies or ideas presented. While this book will be helpful, it is not therapy. If you need further support, please use the code below to open a website that links to mental health resources in your country, including counselling phone lines (available 24 hours a day) and pathways to find a mental health professional.

You are not alone. Support is available.
Reach out early and often.

Self-care

Old rule

Self-care means
putting yourself first.

New rule

'Us-care' means when
we care for others,
we care for ourselves.

‘*Just do more self-care.*’ These days, it feels like self-care is the answer to everything. If you are stressed, anxious or not coping, it's because you aren't doing enough self-care, and if you just did more you would feel better.

Now, it's true that a focus on self-care may be exactly what you need. For the black and queer activists who brought the term into culture in the 1970s–80s, self-care was about knowing your worth in a society where you were not treated as equal. It was about looking after yourself so you could maintain the ability to care for the community.

This was the type of self-care that self-described 'black, lesbian, mother, warrior, poet' Audre Lorde was referring to when she wrote, 'caring for myself is not self-indulgence, it is self-preservation, and that is an act of political warfare'.[3] Self-care asks you to revolt against the expectations of others and put yourself first; to know that you are worthy of care, and through this knowledge build a self-worth that becomes the foundation to wellbeing.

And while the concept of self-care is helpful if it gives you permission to rise against expectations and live life defined by what you need, as I look through my Instagram feed, it seems the term has come to represent something different. Less political warfare, more #selfcare.

To begin with, I think self-care has become too focused on self.

Firstly, if you only focus on self, you start to view self-care as something that is a solo effort. Something you buy for yourself. Or something you do alone to make yourself feel better. But that may mean you don't consider that many of the worthwhile actions of self-care are carried out in relation to other people, such as communicating boundaries, saying no, or standing up for yourself.

Secondly, a focus only on self can leave little room to consider external factors, which can make self-care difficult. I see the impact of this when people start to feel shame for the self-care they are not doing, because rather than considering all the factors that are acting against us, we blame ourselves. The concept of self-care becomes counter-productive when it starts to feel like another thing we are failing at.

It is also useful to consider how self-care is part of an overarching perspective, especially in Western cultures, which views mental health problems as existing within individuals and places responsibility on the individual to fix them. You are diagnosed with a disorder, and you should practise mindfulness, take medication, or go to therapy (the list goes on) to get better. We are told to focus on making ourselves better without considering the health of the community around us. In many ways, this is the logical outcome of a Western culture grounded in individualism: the idea that freedom of thought and action for each person is the most important quality of a society, rather than shared effort and responsibility.[4] The unfortunate by-product of the belief that 'I can do anything' is the self-critical thought that 'my problems are my fault'.

If you are a member of a dominant group – e.g., heterosexual, white, male, and/or able-bodied – a focus on individual responsibility may not seem like an unhelpful idea. For example, although I am queer, I am also able-bodied, white, and male, so, as far as the privilege ladder goes, I'm high up the rungs. Therefore, in many ways, a focus on individual responsibility for my mental health seems useful, because generally – and this is one of the most privileged things you will ever hear a person say – it feels like the only thing standing in my way is myself.

But your experience, especially if you are a member of one or more minority groups, may be vastly different. Standing between you and self-care may be many systemic barriers: racism every time you leave the house, sexism when you try to put yourself first, ableism when you ask for what you need, or transphobia when you are just trying to live your life. This is exhausting and makes self-care harder. And self-care culture may not validate these challenges, but rather tell you to 'just do it' and 'you've got this'.

The unfortunate by-product of the belief that 'I can do anything' is the self-critical thought that 'my problems are my fault'.

Self-care as a distraction

Imagine you had to go and see a psychologist or therapist right now. What would you expect them to be able to do for you? What would you want to get out of these sessions?

I find people mostly come to see me because they want practical strategies that will help alleviate difficult emotions – e.g., to relieve anxiety, anger, or stress. This is because, although we may know we are unhappy in our relationships and unfulfilled with work, we don't often view changing our relationships or job as the way to help. Rather, we want someone to make us feel better about our current choices. We want to learn how to make ourselves feel better about our lives as they are, because we've convinced ourselves that changing our lives is not possible.

I think this is the narrative that self-care feeds into. Self-care can become a distraction from big change that may be needed in your life. This is especially true when we look outside of ourselves for what type of self-care we 'should' be doing – desperately hoping to find the yoga class, breathing exercise or meditation that will make us feel better about our lives and where the world is headed. But if self-care is helping you cope with something that you should change, then this is not self-care – this is self-neglect.

No amount of listening to a mindfulness app is going to make you feel better about a job that you hate. Writing down something you are grateful for should not help you become happy in a bad relationship. If self-care isn't working, it's probably because you need to make a change to your life. Self-care becomes dysfunctional when it distracts you from your needs and demanding better from society.

However, the wellness industry (and it has become an industry) would have us believe that self-care is only about adding small actions to your day that make you feel good. But to improve our mental health, we often need to take actions or make decisions that do not feel good in the moment, even though they are needed. Good mental health requires us to take vulnerable and necessary action that changes the way we live and how we are showing up in our relationships, and work consistently to make significant changes to how we live.

'You can't pour from an empty cup' is an analogy often used when discussing self-care. The idea is that everything we do each day empties our cup. So, from Instagram to sessions with our psychologist, we are encouraged to 'fill up our cup' through self-care. But sometimes the reason your cup keeps emptying is because it's broken. If you put all your time and energy into filling your cup, you may be missing the point. You may need to find the leak and mend it. Or, maybe, you need a new cup.

Self-care becomes dysfunctional when it distracts you from your needs and demanding better from society.

Big change

What might life look like if, rather than focusing on little additions of self-care practices, you take a step back and consider what big changes are needed in your life?

Now when I say big change, I don't mean a long-term goal. The type of big change I'm asking you to consider is something you can do in the short term that shifts your life significantly. Not a dream of what you want your life to become, but an action that takes a step toward it. This might look like quitting a job, starting study, ending a relationship, or moving overseas. It's not a small step, it's a leap.

Now, if even just thinking about the big change needed in your life is difficult, don't fear, you are not alone. This anxiety is just the normal outcome of the evolution of the human brain.

Your brain has evolved to predict threat. The prehistoric person who was focused on risk and looking out for potential danger was more likely to survive. Therefore, your brain has evolved to have an aversion to making big changes, because it is focused on perceiving those changes as threatening and dangerous. Our brains have a bias to focus on avoidance of immediate discomfort and are terrible at keeping focus on the long-term benefits of big change.

So, while the anxious mind is great at protecting you from being trampled by a woolly mammoth, it's not going to get you the life you want. To do that, we need to hijack your brain (just a little). We can show your brain that short-term risks are not the only risks to be aware of. We can point our anxious mind towards another risk – one that we tend to avoid talking about but that, when harnessed, can lead to immense change in our lives.

○

Let's talk about death, baby

Here's something you weren't expecting to read today: you need to start thinking more about your death. All that time and energy you are spending trying to avoid thinking about it is cutting you off from the greatest motivator of all: the knowledge that your life is finite.

Think about it this way: if you found out you were going to die in 12 months, how would you change your life?

See, death is the ultimate motivator. While the avoidance of death stagnates our motivation, as we feel everything can just be done in the future, a focus on death can motivate us to make change in our lives. Big change. Right now.

If you put all your time and energy into filling your cup, you may be missing the point. You may need to find the leak and mend it. Or, maybe, you need a new cup.

Psychologists refer to this as mortality salience and put it forward as one of the reasons people have been making big changes in their lives after the challenges of the pandemic.[5] For many of us, this time brought us face to face with death more than ever before. Whether you were grieving the death of a loved one or feeling connected to the immense grief around the world, thinking about death was unavoidable. One response to acknowledging the inevitability of death is to examine your own life in a new way. We may become more motivated to make significant change if the possibility we may die tomorrow seems more real.

This is what existentialist psychologists like Irvin Yalom invite us to consider: 'though the physicality of death destroys us, the idea of death may save us'.[6] If just reading this section has got you feeling anxious, Yalom would invite you to see that anxiety as useful, because it is a motivator to change. The way through this is not to get rid of your anxiety, but to make your life better now, as 'the more unlived your life, the greater your death anxiety'.[7]

Us-care

We need to reconsider not the intention of self-care, but what the culture has become. The wellness industry has encouraged a culture that is grounded in purchasing self-care for yourself. Therefore, it has capitalised on the idea that you should prioritise your own needs. Through this definition, putting yourself first starts to become viewed against the needs of others. A binary is set up: self-care versus caring for others.

But this binary does not account for perhaps the most beneficial actions for wellbeing – those that benefit self and others. Those that benefit 'us'.

I use the term 'us' here purposefully because I want to use a term that invites you to consider you and the people in your life as one. To consider how the actions you take to care for yourself impact others, and how the actions you take to care for others impact you. The focus on the 'individual' that self-care has encouraged can lead to the belief that when you are doing things for our community or your family, you are only doing something for others. But you're not; you're doing something that impacts you, as well as your people. The choices you make in life impact your 'us'.

This is certainly not a new idea. It is the foundation of many collectivist cultures, including Aboriginal and Torres Strait Islander peoples. Within the oldest continuous living cultures in the world, kinship and the health of your community are viewed as central to wellbeing.[8] Such an understanding of wellbeing invites us to ask the question, why should we view ourselves as healthy, if our community is sick?

Further, a focus on self-care can distract from the power of individuals to contribute to a collective that, together, can make change that can impact the health of that collective. When you start to view wellbeing through an understanding of how your actions impact 'us', you can start to see how self-care may distract you from the changes needed in society and the benefits that may be found through a focus on community. If we only focus on ourselves, who is going to help change the world?

I was tempted here to point to research that shows that doing things for other people is good for your wellbeing, but, ultimately, I think that encourages the same binary. Acts of kindness for others are viewed as something you are doing for someone else. But this is an outcome of individualism that we can choose to step away from, to focus instead on an understanding of wellbeing grounded in the collective, to encourage behaviour that benefits not only the community, but also you, as part of that community. This is important to consider in the context of loneliness and isolation intensified by the pandemic. If you do not feel connected to others, then actions can only be understood within the binary of self-care and care for others.

We must develop a wellbeing culture that supports individuals to look after themselves, while also encouraging people to realise that actions taken to improve community wellbeing help them too. We can encourage a perspective that views poor mental health not as a problem within individuals, but as an indicator that systemic change is needed.

Perhaps this is something that we can take from the last few years: that big change is possible not only in our lives, but in the systems that surround us. In response to the pandemic, massive changes were made to systems overnight. Businesses allowed flexible work arrangements, some for the first time. Events started being presented online, increasing accessibility for people with disability. Governments increased income support payments that saved lives. In Australia, the increase in payments to low-income and unemployed families pulled thousands of children out of poverty. This is not to say the pandemic didn't bring devastating challenges and a staggering loss of life, but it shows us that massive changes to the structures and systems that define society are possible. We just need to be motivated to make the change and, as a collective, demand it.

Nothing matters

I have recently noticed a growing nihilism among friends, clients, and myself; a sense that life had lost meaning. Beyond apathy, it's more a hopelessness. 'What's the point of working or studying if I'm never going to be able to afford a house?' 'What's the point of caring about anything if no one is doing anything about climate change?'

Perhaps, though, we could look at this another way: if the universe and everything has no purpose, then you get to dictate what the purpose is.

This has been termed 'optimistic nihilism'.[9] This idea proposes that we should accept that we are all going to die - that the universe is going to end; that none of the social norms matter; that nothing matters. It allows us to take away all rules and expectations. So then what are we left with?

We are left with ourselves, and the people and the environment around us.

And perhaps this is where the focus can be: considering your actions based on what they do for you, your community, and the environment. And understanding how your actions contribute not only to your own wellbeing, but also to the wellbeing of your community.

When we only focus on the self, the actions we take seem insignificant against the epic problems the world is facing. But if we widen our view to see how our 'little' actions are being repeated and amplified by others, we can feel a greater sense of power and optimism for change. Staying focused on the knowledge that our actions are part of a greater collective contribution makes a difference; knowing that we are part of a long history of people and, together, we make change.

Perhaps the answer to nihilism and hopelessness in the world cannot only be self-care, but a focus on community.

We need to move away from a culture that views self-care as the end goal, and a wellness industry that sells us the path to get there. Rather, we need to acknowledge that the end goal here is a meaningful life. And the actions that lead to a life of meaning are a lot less about buying stuff, and a lot more about boundaries and belonging. They are actions of saying no, being vulnerable, making big changes, and being connected to the people around you. And none of these actions requires you to purchase anything. Self-care may be the first step towards a meaningful life, but it is not the last.

Self-care may
be the first
step towards a
meaningful life,
but it is not
the last.

New rules in action • New rules in action •

Redefining self-care

Self-care becomes unhelpful when it becomes focused on looking outward to external expectations of what good self-care should be, rather than turning inward to understand what you need.

A good starting point can be to regularly take a self-care stocktake, giving yourself a score out of 10 for how well you are caring for yourself across each of these five self-care domains: sleep (quantity and quality), movement (whatever that looks like for you), connection (with the important people in your life), nourishment, and pleasure. And for those domains with the lowest scores, consider what actions could increase the score, even just a little. You can also focus on redefining self-care through asking yourself these questions daily:

1. How can I care for myself today?

2. What are the barriers to making that happen? Can they be challenged?

3. What can I do to help make that care happen?

4. What positive impact will this care have not only for me, but for my community and the people in my life?

Us-care

Defining your 'us'

1. Write a list of all the important people in your life, including family, friends and colleagues.

2. Write a list of the collectives or groups you are part of.

3. Imagine these people all together. What emotions does it bring up for you to imagine being in that space with them all? This is your 'us'.

Us actions

1. Write a list of 5–10 achievable actions that would benefit your 'us' – i.e., they would benefit you as well as the people you care about.

2. Focus on one action. Write a few sentences about why this action would be meaningful for your 'us', and why it would be meaningful for you.

3. When you complete the action, consider if the action had the intended impact. A different impact? An impact you might not be aware of?

4. Consider if your action may have contributed to a greater purpose; try to see the action as part of a change, rather than 'the change'.

Let's get impractical

Okay, let's take some time to play around with some ideas of the big change you want to see in your life. And I use the word 'play' here with purpose, because I want this to feel like fun – because, if you're like me, you've stopped being good at play and you've become good at planning. Planning is the writing down and thinking about the how. The steps it will take to achieve something. The practical things. Although this is helpful, that's not what we are doing now. If we are going to make big change, we are going to need to think big, use our imagination and get creative.

1. Take a sheet of blank paper and a pen (if you love stationery, this is the chance to get out the good stuff).

2. Take 5 deep breaths and start a 20-minute timer.

   * Write down some of the big ideas for change you want to see in your life. The big, audacious goals. Dreams. You may also like to use some other creative means to explore this, like painting or drawing.

   * As difficult emotions come up, observe the emotions with compassion and curiosity. Remind yourself they are a normal part of the process.

   * Notice when your brain starts thinking about the planning or the reasons why something cannot happen, and move your attention back to play and creativity.

3. After 20 minutes, consider what you have written down. How does it feel to look at the list?

Making big change happen

Okay, looking at your list of dreams, choose one to focus on. Now try to think of a big change in your life that could help make that dream happen. Remember, a big change is not a long-term goal; it's an action that you can do in the short term that starts a big change in your life.

1. Write down one big change and answer the following questions:

   * Why is this important to you?

   * Why is this important for your 'us'?

   * What could help you achieve this?

   * What are the difficult emotions that come up when you think about this change, and are likely to come up as you act on this change? Are you willing to allow space for these emotions to make this change?

   * What are the short-term risks that your brain is focusing on? What are the meaningful long-term gains that your brain is not focusing on?

2. Write a list of the possible positive and negative outcomes of this decision. And, because each outcome will have a different level of impact on your life, give each a rating out of 5 (high scores meaning the outcome would make a big difference in your life). Compare the scores for each column.

3. If you are ready to commit to the change, hijack your brain's bias towards avoidance of short-term discomfort by carrying a note in your phone or wallet that shows all the long-term gains to be made by making a big change. Pull out this list and look at it when you feel like not following through with this action.

Emotions

Old rule

Emotions should
be controlled.

New rule

Emotions should
be understood with
openness and curiosity.

Crying. **This is how you started life – freely expressing your emotions, letting the world know how you were feeling. And the people around you responded to this emotion.**

But then life happened. Family, friends, and society started teaching us about our emotions, the meaning we should give them and how we should respond to them. We came to learn that many of our emotions should be experienced in private and expressed with caution.

We learned that some emotions are 'good' and some are 'bad'. And that if we are experiencing a bad one, we should do all we can to get rid of it, avoid it, or at least distract ourselves from it.

We learned that some emotions can be expressed, but only in certain circumstances, with certain people. When asked how we are feeling, we should say 'good'. If we are not feeling up to work or other responsibilities, we should disconnect from our emotions and push through.

We learned not to talk about our emotions, and because of that, no one honestly talks about how they are feeling. And because of that, we think that we are the only ones who feel like this.

We learned that if we are feeling tired, we should drink coffee. If we are feeling sad, we should take a pill. Our anger needs management. Our excitement is too much. Our jealousy is ridiculous. Our fear is unwarranted. And our anxiety is pathological.

We are told that we are too emotional, and that this is a bad thing.

A battle begins – a conflict between how we feel inside, and the person we must be in the world. Our emotions are viewed as something that gets in the way of life, something to be managed so we can just get on with it.

And the field of psychology is as much to blame as anything else. We sell therapy that aims to reduce emotion, to alleviate depression or anxiety. We, as much as anyone, perpetuate the idea that our emotions are symptoms that need to be treated and controlled.

Now, I need to be clear here: therapy helps. People who experience mental illness should seek help. But, in my experience, therapy does not work by reducing emotion (in fact, I have many clients who see me because they feel disconnected from their emotions and want to get that feeling back). Therapy works when it teaches skills that allow emotions to be processed and validated so that they become part of our lives, instead of controlling our lives. The emotions don't go away; they just become something that is observed, something to make space for.

Indeed, I find the sooner we stop wishing we felt better, paradoxically, the sooner we feel better.

It's not about feeling better; it's about getting better at feeling.

Standing in the way of control

Perhaps the most unhelpful rule we learn in life is that we can and must control our emotions. If our emotions are overwhelming, we just need to find the right strategy; if we do it enough, the emotions will go away, and we can get back to life.

We try to control them but fail. This is because you can't control emotions - they are not a malfunction; they are a normal physiological system of the human body.

To help understand this, let's take another system of the body: breathing. Imagine if, when you were young, your friends and your family told you to stop breathing in public - that you breathe too much. Imagine being told that little boys don't breathe and that little girls can breathe, but only in specific ways. So, you try to breathe only if you absolutely have to. You hide your breathing in public. You hold your breath for extended periods of time. But the need to breathe grows stronger. And eventually you must breathe. And then you get frustrated with yourself for breathing because you should have been able to control it like everyone else. And this cycle continues because you need to breathe.

Obviously, that sounds ridiculous, and no one would ever ask anyone to stop breathing - to stop using a system of the body that is vital for survival. But that's exactly what disconnecting from your emotions is. Because your emotions are also vital for survival.

Repeatedly you are asked to shut down or ignore this vital system and to cut off from the reality of your emotions, even though the recognition, understanding, and expression of emotions is one of the most important physiological systems we have. It helps us make sense of the world, understand the environment around us, notice threat, build social connections, and understand the needs of others. This is why we should trust our gut, as our emotions tell us the right thing to do when we cognitively just can't work it out. No matter how hard we try to ignore, distract, or control our emotions, we can't, because emotions are vital.

This is the first step to accepting and developing openness to emotion - understanding that emotions are not a threat, because they are part of you.

Perhaps we could understand this like we understand pain. Pain, at its core, is an emotion. It is something we feel. Pain is our body's signal that something isn't right. If we numb it or distract ourselves from it, we miss the opportunity to get a better understanding of the pain and what is causing it. We need to see all emotions in this way, as temporary states that should be understood, not ignored. It's not about feeling better; it's about getting better at feeling.

So how do we get better at feeling? We need to take time to make meaning of the physical state of emotion, rather than attempt to numb or avoid it, or struggle as we try to control it.

Psychologist Susan David describes this as skills in 'emotional agility'.[10] David's work invites us to use our emotions and thoughts as important sources of information, but not to allow them to overwhelm us and take our attention away from living by our values. As David describes, 'thoughts and emotions contain information, not direction'.[11]

We can't control our emotions, but we can change our attitude towards them. Although challenging and hard-won, the ability to stay present while noticing your emotions with an attitude of curiosity and openness is key.

Let me repeat this, for it is one of the most useful ideas I will ever impart: the key to wellbeing is the ability to turn toward your emotions with compassionate curiosity rather than a want to control.

Unfortunately, your brain is not a helpful ally in this quest for curiosity. I'm sure you've noticed this – your brain does not deal well with uncertainty. And curiosity is all about moving towards uncertainty with openness and interest.

Your brain desperately, and effortfully, wants to categorise and predict your life. Your brain takes short cuts. If I asked how you are feeling, your brain doesn't want to take the time and effort to examine how you are feeling, so we pick an umbrella term. Stressed. Anxious. Angry. Tired. This is a problem, because the language we attach to our emotions changes our experience of them.[12]

A limited emotion vocabulary can limit our experience – our partner makes us 'angry', we are 'stressed' at work, and feel 'tired' all the time. If we focus on these umbrella terms, we may miss the meaning that can be found through naming the specific emotion that hides beneath. In reality you may be fearful that your partner doesn't love you anymore, or disappointed that you are in a job you don't find meaningful.

Through this lens we can come to understand that underneath a lack of motivation or confidence are often specific emotions that need to be processed – e.g., feeling overwhelmed, fearful, or helpless. Such specific labelling of your emotions not only changes your experience of them but allows for more useful behaviour based on this specific understanding. It allows you to listen to your emotions in the way they are intended; it helps you create meaning from the world around you.

To our brains, a perceived certainty is far easier to process than the uncertain reality of life. And the fact of the matter is, we live in an uncertain reality. Although significant challenges such as the COVID-19 pandemic, climate crisis, and rising geopolitical tensions may lead us to desperately seek the solace of certainty, the hard truth is that it's never going to come. Simply because we can't predict the future.

The alternative is to focus on observing the present in all its uncomfortable glory. But this is scary. It means sitting in the vulnerability and ambiguity of life. But the more we do this, the more opportunity we create for something phenomenal to happen. We will start to see the true value of emotions, because our emotions are the system that helps us make sense of the present. Our emotions give us precise, moment-to-moment information about our environment and our place in it. Emotions tell us if we are under threat, help us empathise with how people around us are feeling, and help us learn what is meaningful to us in life. Our emotions help us make sense of the uncertainty. But only if we tune in to them and listen.

The key to wellbeing is the ability to turn toward your emotions with compassionate curiosity rather than a want to control.

Stress is a process

When I feel stressed, my initial response is to consume something to distract me from the feeling. Chocolate, TV and wine are my go-tos. For a short while this works, but then the stress returns, often even stronger than before.

When those tactics fail, I might try talking about my stress. Well, let's be honest, when I say 'talking about my stress', I mean complaining about the cause of my stress. Although this helps a little, I often leave these conversations unsettled, heightened and, well ... stressed.

Then, like a good psychologist should, I might notice my anxious thoughts. I write them down. Challenge them. I try to say something I'm grateful for. I think about what a friend would say to me right now. I'm a psychologist, remember – I know a technique or two.

After all this, I'm still stressed. Why? Because I haven't done anything to process the emotion. My body wants to run and fight, but I'm not letting it.

We can spend so much time talking about stress that we forget that it is a normal response of the human body. And the better we can understand the stress response, the better we can manage our mental health. The first step is understanding stress as a process.

Go time

The process starts when your amygdala (the
emotional centre of your brain) perceives a threat.
This might be something in the environment that's
a real threat to your safety (for example, a bear),
or something your frontal lobe has just imagined
is a threat (for example, an overdue essay about
bears). Either way, the amygdala signals to the
hypothalamus that it is go time – imagine the
hypothalamus like a driver who has the options to
accelerate or brake.

When your brain perceives a threat, the
accelerator is on, and your sympathetic nervous
system (which controls your body's response
to danger or stress) kicks into gear, pumping
adrenaline and cortisol to get your body into the
famous 'fight-or-flight' mode. The heart rate rises,
muscles get more blood, breath becomes more rapid,
senses become sharper, and nutrients flood the
bloodstream. Your body is prepared for the threat.[13]

Now if there is a real threat (like the bear) you
would run or fight, just as your body has evolved
to do. However, these days often the source of your
stress is not something you can fight or run away
from – a global pandemic, the thought you are going
to fail, a guy who hasn't messaged back, or the fear of
your partner leaving you.

And if our body can't complete the stress cycle, we get stuck in it. In the words of Emily and Amelia Nagoski, authors of *Burnout*, 'Stress is not bad for you; being stuck is bad for you.'[14]

The excellent Emily and Amelia remind us that we often stay stuck in the stress because we don't use strategies based in the body. We focus on strategies that try to distract us from the stress, rather than process it. Or we ruminate on the cause of the stress, even though it's outside of our control.

It must be said that if you can take action to change the thing causing the stress, you should. But when you can't, it can be incredibly helpful to instead focus on completing the stress cycle.

Finishing the race

Remember your sympathetic response is your foot on the accelerator, so one option is to get to the finish line and let your body complete the cycle. This requires listening to your body and what it needs to do. When you're feeling angry or ready to fight, try vigorous exercise or punching a pillow. When feeling fear, anxiety or a need to escape, try going for a run or cycle outside. This will trick your system into thinking it has taken action to protect itself against the threat. And once the body has done that, it can relax. Literally.

Anxiety is not a problem that exists within us; it is a cycle we need to change.

Putting on the brakes

So far, I have only described the accelerator, the sympathetic nervous system. But luckily your body also has a brake: the parasympathetic nervous system. This is the system that promotes calm and relaxation: less 'fight or flight', more 'rest and digest'. The major nerve of this system is the vagus nerve, which, when stimulated, will lead the body to feel safe.[15] And because the brain monitors the body, you will start to perceive yourself as safe. These are exactly the skills you can use if there is an environment or object that your brain perceives as threatening, even though you know it to be safe – e.g., social situations, flying on a plane, etc.

Changing the cycle

Anxiety is not a problem that exists within us; it is a cycle we need to change – an interaction between your environment, your perception of that environment and your body's reaction. The cycle that maintains anxiety disorders is one of avoidance: your brain perceives an environment as threatening, you feel anxious, you perceive the anxiety as threatening, you avoid it, and the anxiety reduces. This would be fine if the aim of life was to avoid anxiety, but it's not. The way you might work with a psychologist to change this cycle is through doing the thing that makes you anxious while using strategies to stimulate the vagus nerve (e.g., deep breathing) and noticing your anxiety is not a threat – it is just a message from your body based on a false perception. Over time your brain will learn that the environment is not a threat to your safety, because it monitors the body.

It is also important to note that you don't have to wait for stress or anxiety to engage the vagus nerve. The more we do this, the more we increase what's called 'vagal tone', which has been shown to not only improve overall wellbeing, lower heart rate and improve digestion, but to also make your sympathetic nervous system less sensitive and your parasympathetic nervous system more likely to engage – i.e., you stress less and relax faster.[16] If that sounds pretty appealing, check out the strategies to engage your vagus nerve on pages 69-71.

Making meaning of discomfort

It can be a challenging experience to notice just how much of our time and energy we give to attempts to distract, avoid, and control emotions.

We avoid conversations that are likely to bring up emotion. We avoid work that is stressful. We reach for our phone the moment we start feeling worried. We have the TV on because it distracts us from the feelings.

Not only do these attempts often lead to negative health consequences, but we miss out on the meaningful life we are avoiding. We avoid the meaningful in favour of the comfortable. And no change comes from comfortable.

We avoid talking about emotions because we think that talking about them causes them. But conversations don't cause emotion. They just allow the emotions that are already being felt to be validated and processed so we can move through them.

This is the outcome of viewing some emotions, such as anxiety, fear, or stress, as 'bad'. We can start to see the presence of these emotions as an indicator that we are doing the wrong thing: that a good life is one where we make choices that make us happy and free of 'bad' emotions.

But here's the thing.

It's the opposite.

Uncomfortable emotions are felt when we are doing something that matters.

We feel anxious as we talk in front of a group because it is important to us that they hear what we have to say. We feel stressed at work because what we do matters. We feel guilt when we do something wrong because we know that's not the kind of person we want to be. We feel anger when someone disrespects us because we deserve respect. We feel enormous grief if we lose someone because we loved that person immensely. Not only do these emotions make sense – they in fact tend to become more intense the more important something is to us.

And with this view, we can gain a new understanding of a word that is often misunderstood: resilience. I have noticed this word become something of a weapon of capitalism. When someone is challenged by work or structural inequalities, they are told that the problem is within them – they just need to be more resilient. This creates a culture where, if you are feeling stressed, burnt out, or overwhelmed by some other emotion, you should do something to get rid of that feeling so you can get back to work.

But this is not resilience, this is dysfunction.

Resilience is not the capacity to control our emotions to meet the expectations of others.

Resilience is the willingness to feel uncomfortable emotions as we do something meaningful.

Resilience is the willingness to feel uncomfortable emotions as we do something meaningful. As described by Susan David, 'courage is not the absence of fear but fear walking'.[17]

   Consider my time during the pandemic. I, like everyone else, experienced a roller-coaster of emotions. The stress, anxiety, and grief of being in the longest lockdown in the world was real. I was feeling it, right alongside my clients. But I kept working. I kept turning on the computer screen, giving therapy to that little green light and supporting clients through significant mental health challenges. But trust me, I did not find some magic way to get rid of my emotions to allow me to do this. I kept focus on why what I was doing was meaningful and validated my emotions. I reminded myself that my fear, grief, and frustration were a normal part of this process. It even became helpful for me to let my clients know that I was suffering too. We could hold space for our grief because we gave it meaning. An emotion ceases to control us the moment we make it meaningful. Suffering is often beyond our control, but our attitude towards that suffering can be the difference between coping and collapse. This is how a marathon runner can push through the pain, a parent can work endlessly to support their children, or you can get up and be there for a friend, even on the days you feel exhausted.

This is what becoming better at feeling looks like. It is noticing our emotional experiences, giving them meaning and reminding ourselves that it's a normal part of the process of living. It's about taking time to process the emotion, so we can move through it.

However, this needs to be more than just an idea. What I've often seen happen, in workshops and in sessions, is that we talk about being open to emotions, but it becomes a theory that is never put into practice. But the skill in recognising, understanding, and making meaning from emotions is a process of unlearning that is only achieved through action (like those in the next section).

Suffering is often beyond our control, but our attitude towards that suffering can be the difference between coping and collapse.

New rules in action • New rules in action •

It is important to consider your intention before using these strategies, as the intention will change the effectiveness of the strategy. If you are using a strategy with the intention to get rid of an emotion, it is very likely that you will become frustrated. Instead, set the intention to make space for emotions, so they become experiences you view with curiosity and can gently observe while you move your attention back to the present.

I also want to acknowledge that while the following skills are shown to be helpful, even in processing difficult emotions, this work can become overwhelming for some people, especially if you have experienced trauma. If this is the case for you, I would suggest working with a trauma-informed mental health professional to learn skills in processing emotion that work best for you (the QR code at the start of the book may be a good place to start).

How to process stress

Physical exertion tends to be the fastest way to process stress, as blood can pump oxygen through the muscles and work out the adrenaline and cortisol through exhaling carbon dioxide and sweat. Listening to your body will be key to working out what you need. When in heightened stress (fight-or-flight response), vigorous exercise might be needed (exercise that breaks a sweat). However, when your stress has become overwhelming towards a freeze response, you might try a hug, stretching, something creative, or a breathing exercise.

How to move through emotion

As emotions arise, your first response may be to distract yourself. Sometimes this is what you need to do. However, sometimes you will have the capacity to understand and process your emotions through the following steps:

1. Take a breath and move your attention to the physical sensation of the emotion in your body. Just notice it with openness and curiosity.

2. Find the right word to label your emotion. Try the feeling wheels (on the next three pages) by starting with the general emotion in the centre, and then moving out to find a label that more precisely describes your experience.

3. Take time to validate your emotion. Ask yourself: 'Why does it makes sense that I feel like this?'

4. Notice if this emotion is directing you to take action or communicating a need, or if you just need to ground yourself (see page 69) as you wait for the emotion to pass.

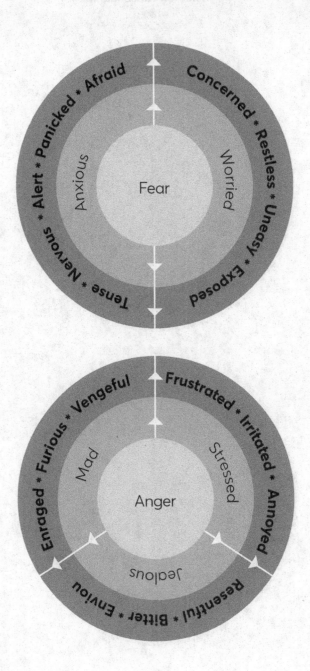

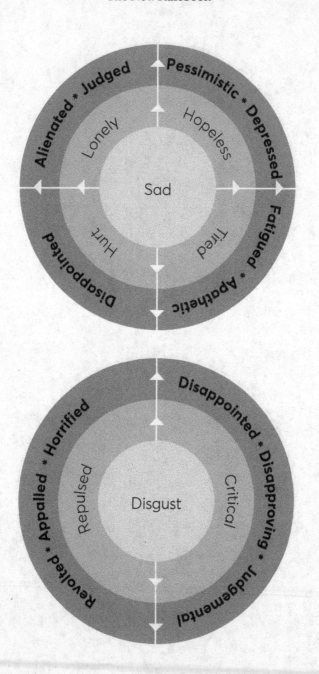

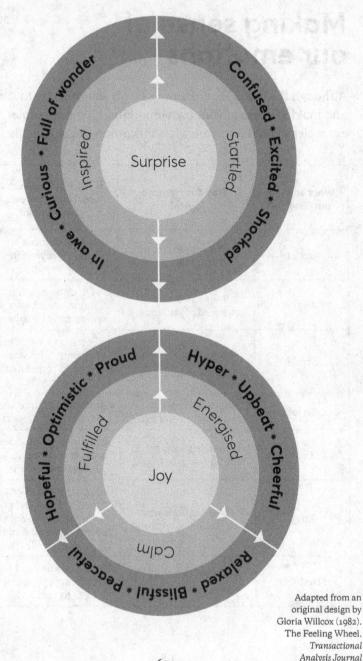

Adapted from an
original design by
Gloria Willcox (1982).
The Feeling Wheel.
*Transactional
Analysis Journal*

Making sense of our emotions

Although the focus should always be on your turning inward and making sense of your own emotions, below are some examples to help illustrate what this process may look like.

What emotion am I feeling?	Why does it make sense?	Is there an action that could help process this emotion?
Anxiety	I am doing something that matters.	I need to focus on grounding myself in the present.
Anger	Someone has not respected my boundary.	Do some vigorous exercise and later reiterate my boundary.
Stress	Something is beyond my control.	Focus on what is in my control. Do some exercise to complete the stress cycle.
Grief	I have suffered a loss of someone meaningful.	Allow myself time and reach out for support.
Fear	I am doing something new and unpredictable.	Just notice the fear and focus on why this action is important to me.
Envy	My partner is away with friends for the weekend.	Breathe and allow myself to feel it. Notice if it is telling me about something I desire more of in my life.
Tiredness	I have been working late and not sleeping well.	Set boundaries and say no to create opportunity to rest.

Getting grounded

When emotions have become overwhelming, the following can be useful in stimulating the vagus nerve and to help you become present. Keep in mind these techniques are not about controlling your emotional state, but rather moving your attention to something else (e.g., your body or your senses) as you allow the emotion to pass.

Deep slow breathing

Although there are many different techniques, the basic premise is to keep your attention with the sensory experience of breathing as you take slow, deep breaths. For more specific guidance you could try the following diaphragmatic breathing technique, which is backed by research as effective in stimulating the vagus nerve.[18]

Prepare: Find somewhere comfortable to sit or lie down. Ensure your back is supported and your feet are firmly on the floor. Place one hand on your chest, the other on your stomach. Gently observe your body. Bring your attention to your breath.

1. Breathe in through your nose, counting to 4 slowly. Notice your stomach rise and the feeling of your body supported.

2. Hold for 4 seconds.

3. Exhale through your mouth for 8 seconds.

4. Repeat for at least 10 breaths, or until you feel grounded.

Mindfulness

This is the process of focusing your attention on the present moment, while gently accepting your emotions, thoughts, and bodily sensations. This might be achieved through a mindfulness exercise led by an app or audio clip. Or try a 'mindful moment', where you keep your attention on the sensations of an action for 3 minutes. For example, drink a glass of water and notice how it tastes and how the glass feels, take a walk and focus on the world around you, or listen to music and try to really hear each instrument.

The five senses exercise

The following can be helpful for yourself or to guide someone else through, if they are feeling panicked, overwhelmed, or disconnected.

- Notice 5 things that you can **see**.
- Notice 4 things that you can **feel**.
- Notice 3 things that you can **hear**.
- Notice 2 things that you can **smell**.
- Notice 1 thing that you can **taste**.

Feet on the ground

Notice where your feet are connected to the ground. It might help to find some grass and take your shoes off to feel your feet on the earth. If you are in a building, close your eyes and imagine how your feet connect to the floor, which connects to the building floor, which, in turn, connects to the earth. Imagine your weight finding grounding through to the earth below.

Using your voice to anchor

Try chanting, singing, gargling, or humming. It might also be helpful to find a phrase to centre you. You may have to practise until you find one that works for you. Some examples include: 'Let it be,' 'This too shall pass,' 'This is a moment of suffering, and suffering is a part of a meaningful life,' 'May I be kind and gentle on myself,' or, one of my favourites from artist and writer Samuel Leighton-Dore, 'I am safe, I am loved, I am sexy.'[19]

Work

Old rule

Work hard and you
will be rewarded.

New rule

Live authentically
with purpose.

Stop setting goals. **Okay, you might not have been expecting to hear that. It might go against every rule you've been taught about getting the life you want. Hell, it might even go against everything your psychologist has said.**

Goals – especially long-term ones – trick you into thinking you are completely in control of your life. But the thing is, you're not.

Think about a goal you have in life. Now take a moment to recognise all the things – the ones beyond your control – that might happen to get in the way of you reaching that goal. If the last few years have taught us anything, it's that life has a way of throwing a lot of unprecedented challenges at us. And with long-term goals, you have pretty much created a structure that ensures you will not be truly happy or satisfied until you achieve your goal, no matter if the path to achieve it has little to do with you.

Think about some goals you have had in the past. Why did you set these goals? Were they meaningful to you or did you just set them because you felt you should?

When I reflect on my life, I can see an exhausting string of goals, each of which took an incredible amount of work to achieve. However, when it really comes down to it, most were more about meeting expectations rather than working towards goals that were meaningful to me.

We often set goals that are not important to us. This is especially true for work, which can feel like an endless list of goals that are given to you, rather than important to you. This is the fine line between goals and expectations. As soon as you lose touch with why a goal is meaningful to you, it ceases to be a goal and becomes an expectation. You may still be motivated to achieve it, but now that motivation tends to be based in fear of failure, the need to please people, or the need to complete it just because you started it. These factors can be incredibly motivating, but as they are based in self-criticism, it can make the journey to the goal a life not worth living. Also, when you achieve the goal, you tend to not care that much, or perhaps not even notice. It doesn't feel like a moment of achievement and satisfaction, but rather only a meeting of expectation.

Just think how much time and energy we spend working towards goals at work and what these goals are motivated by. I mean, if an alien came down to Earth and was asked to infer what the meaning of life was for human beings, after not too long I'm pretty sure our alien friend would say 'money'.

Now if you don't like this summation (and I'm right there with you), what would you prefer that alien to report back? Imagine what human life could achieve if we stopped putting so much of our energy towards the pursuit of work and money. What could life look like?

But that's a big question. Let's look at something a little closer to home. Imagine an alien came to Earth and had to observe your behaviour for a week. What would they conclude is most important in your life? What is most of your behaviour motivated by? How do you spend most of your time?

Now, if the answers to that are a little alarming, don't worry. I've got a new path you might like to consider.

○

Who are you?

Complete the following sentence and feel free to use a few words:

I am a ...

Perhaps you wrote something about your role in your family (e.g., mother or father), your gender, sexuality, or some other aspect of your identity. I've done this with hundreds of people and I find many of us write something else. Something to do with our work.

Somewhere along the way, our work becomes enmeshed with who we are. It becomes our identity.

As soon as you
lose touch with
why a goal is
meaningful to you,
it ceases to be a
goal and becomes
an expectation.

And this may mean we start to assess our worth based on our productivity, achievement, or salary. And within a capitalist society, this mindset fits quite nicely. But just because it's the norm doesn't mean it is functional.

If work has become your identity, it makes sense that it gets all your attention because it has become the way to earn self-worth. But you are not your work. It is something you do. Your work is an important part of your identity, but it is not the only thing that defines you. Work is not who you are, work is a place where you can enact who you are.

But if your worth is not going to be determined by your success at work, what is the alternative?

Before we go further, I just want to acknowledge reality for a second. Many of us must work to live. And depending on your situation, it can feel like you need to work to survive. If this is what work feels like for you, I do not want this section to feel like a pressure to quit your job and focus on something 'more meaningful'. Instead, I hope to encourage a mindset that allows you to connect to the meaning in your work, as well as all the other parts of your life. To know your work is meaningful exactly because of the life it allows you to provide for yourself and others. And that is just the beginning.

It's your party

Imagine it's your 80th birthday. You are having a fabulous party because you, and your 80 years on Earth, are certainly worth celebrating. Imagine as you look around that you see everyone from your life. Imagine what food is being served. What music is playing? Close your eyes and picture it.

Then the music stops and someone very important to you appears from the crowd. They walk on to a stage. And give a speech about your life.

How do you want them to describe you? What do you want them to say about the way you have treated people in your life? What words do you want them to use to describe what you have held as most meaningful and important in your life?

These words are your values.

This is a task (check out 'Who Am I?' on page 105) often used in acceptance and commitment therapy[20], and it is one I continue to return to as it really helps people get down to the heart of what a meaningful life is for them – it's also a bit cheerier than a task that gets you to write your own eulogy.

However, over the years I have also noticed that 'values' have got a bit of a bad reputation. Even to the point where I've spent a ridiculous amount of time trying to come up with another term, just to avoid the V word. I think perhaps it's because you've been through one too many meetings at work that have focused on the 'values' of the company. Or in high school you sat through some sort of class where you had to define your values – and that class was boring. Or perhaps you've walked away from workshops with psychologists like me with a sense of what your values were, and it felt good to think about them. But perhaps that's about where it stopped.

You see, values are useless if they just remain an ideal. Values should never be viewed as something to work towards in the future. Your values should feel like something that you can live by every day, no matter the circumstances. As eloquently defined by doctor, psychotherapist and author of *The Happiness Trap*, Russ Harris: 'Values are not the destination. Values are the compass.'[21] To put it another way, we need to spend less time talking about our values, and more time using them to direct a life of purpose.

This connects to a branch of psychology that has emerged in recent years that is all about getting a meaningful life – a movement referred to as positive psychology. And yes, if positive psychology is a new movement, it does suggest that before it there was some sort of 'negative' psychology. To be honest, this is not far from the truth. Psychological theory and research for decades effectively aimed to define what was 'abnormal' and how to support people back to 'normal'. We spent a lot of time focused on what could go wrong in your mental health and how to treat you, and not much time on how to help people be happy. Which, it turns out, is a complex endeavour.

Happiness is not an emotion

As you can imagine, when it comes to defining what makes people happy, things get complicated – as they should. We humans are beautifully complex. To begin with, we must try to define happiness, which is a difficult task. The thing most researchers agree on is that happiness is not just a feeling and that we shouldn't see it as something to aim for, but rather a possible by-product of our actions. They also tend to agree that happiness is made up of two main components. As summarised by positive psychology researcher Sonja Lyubomirsky, happiness is 'the experience of joy, contentment, or positive wellbeing, combined with a sense that one's life is good, meaningful, and worthwhile'.[22] In psychology research, these two components of happiness or, as it is defined in psychology, 'subjective wellbeing' are referred to as hedonic and eudaimonic wellbeing. And these are helpful to examine because, to be happy, we must do both.

Hedonic wellbeing is all about pleasure, enjoyment and life satisfaction.[23] I love this focus, because it reminds us that while we can't make ourselves happy, we sometimes forget that we can do things that are likely to bring on joy and pleasure. And in a culture so focused on work and productivity, fun and desire can be seen as a distraction, or something just for special occasions. But fun and pleasure are central to wellbeing and must be prioritised.

Life satisfaction is also core to hedonic wellbeing. Here it is useful to consider that your ability to feel happiness is not just dependent on feeling joy, but whether you view something as 'enough'. Related to this, psychologists define two mindsets through which people approach life, which impact their ability to be satisfied. So let's find out, are you a maximiser or a satisficer?

Consider the last time you chose somewhere to stay on a holiday. If you are a satisficer, you would have decided on what you needed from the accommodation, booked the first hotel that fit that criterion, and been satisfied with the choice. However, if you kept searching and searching, comparing every choice for maximum benefit, you're a maximiser.[24] And while it might seem like putting time into finding the choice that gives maximum benefit might lead to the most satisfying decision, numerous studies show that this is not the case.[25] Maximisers spend so much energy trying to make the optimal choice that they spend less time appreciating what they have. They also tend to end up dissatisfied with the choice, as they always feel like they could have done better. Happiness doesn't come from making the optimal choice - happiness comes from being satisfied with the choice that fits your needs.

We need to stop focusing on how we live and start focusing on why.

To increase our eudaimonic wellbeing, we must focus on growth, authenticity, meaning, and excellence.[26] This shows us that happiness is achieved through experiences of meaning and purpose. We need to stop focusing on how we live and start focusing on why. So, to be happy we must work out what is authentically meaningful to us and then do it.

That's it. Easy, right?

Absolutely not.

○

Living the good life

You don't need me to tell you what a meaningful life looks like, but you may need me to give you some ideas on how to achieve it. Because it's one thing to imagine your 80th birthday, but it's another thing to make a meaningful life happen. What I find more important than defining your values is understanding the barriers that exist, which act against you living a meaningful life. So, let's examine each of these barriers closely and take our time. After all, we are attempting to define the meaning of life here.

Authenticity requires vulnerability

Authenticity is a two-part process. The first, an internal process, is the ability to know yourself and what you want from life. The second is to put this into action.

I have sat with many people while they attempt to work out this first part of the process, so I know it's not easy. It's very common for people to say at the start of this journey, 'I don't know what I want from life.'

At points like these in therapy I am often reminded of a scene from a therapy session from pioneer family therapist Virginia Satir. A mother is positioned between her husband and her adolescent son, with each taking one of her arms to signify the way she feels pulled between them. At one point Virginia turns to the son and asks:

'What do you want for your mother?'

The son responds, 'For her to have peace of mind.'

Virginia then asks, 'And what do you want for yourself?'

The son pauses. Confused. 'Pertaining to what?'

To which Virginia replies: 'I don't know what you want for yourself, love; what do you want for yourself?'

I think this question best sums up the first step towards authenticity: what do you want for yourself?

This is where things start to feel vulnerable. Although on paper it might seem like naming what is meaningful to you should be a process of joy and hope, actually it is often a process that brings on overwhelming and complex emotions. Often when we compare our imagined meaningful life to the life we are living, we can feel regret for the choices we didn't make, guilt for mistakes we have made, or anger that we have wasted so much of our life on things that do not matter. Uncomfortable emotions are not only a normal part of living a meaningful life, but they are also a normal part of the process of defining what a meaningful life could look like.

The second part of this process of authenticity is to externalise this internal understanding of what you want for your life – to put into action that which is meaningful to you. The vulnerability here is different, as doing what is meaningful is often viewed as a risk, because it goes against the expectations of the people around you and the parts of your mind that tell you what your life 'should' be.

Knowing what is meaningful to you requires unlearning

As soon we start the process of naming our values and putting them into action, there is a common roadblock. The values are clear, the reasons why an action is meaningful are clear, and the path to achieve it is clear. However, when it comes to doing it, there is a common response that stops behaviour change dead in its tracks:

'I can't ... because I must ...'

Every step towards meaningful action becomes viewed as a step away from a responsibility, or expectation, or something else you must do.

Rational emotive behaviour therapy pioneer, Albert Ellis, had a name for this: musterbation.[27] For Ellis, our focus on thoughts that tell us we 'must' do something is always irrational. Further, these beliefs about what we 'must' do are often not based on our current needs but are an outcome of early childhood experiences. To understand this, we need to take a crash course in cognitive behavioural therapy and, specifically, schema therapy.

Schema therapy is a school of therapy introduced by Jeff Young in 1990 that pretty much tried to pull together the best parts of some of the major theories we have in helping people: cognitive behavioural therapy, gestalt therapy, attachment theory, and psychoanalysis – like pulling the best players from multiple teams, each with different strengths, to form a national team.[28] Or, if sporting metaphors aren't your thing, it's like getting Mariah, Whitney, Britney and Gaga together to form a supergroup.

Now what this therapy proposes is that we are all born with basic emotional needs, for affection, guidance, love, shelter and safety, and deficits in how these needs were met in childhood can lead to ways of interpreting the world and the people around you that are not helpful (termed maladaptive schemas). These schemas are understood to be like underlying mindsets, outside of our consciousness, that lead to unhelpful automatic thoughts and coping styles. Here are some common schemas that might be getting in the way of you living a life of meaning:

1. If your caregivers were critical of you or you observed your caregivers being critical of others, you may have developed a self-critical schema. Your attempts to live by values are met with thoughts of 'I will never succeed,' 'It's not worth trying,' or 'Why try? It's just not going to work out for me.'

2. If as a child you were discouraged from doing things alone or were never empowered to be independent, you may have developed a schema of dependence and incompetence. This means attempts to put your values into practice are thwarted by the belief that you cannot trust yourself or achieve things on your own.

3. When your development has involved excessive emotional involvement and closeness with one or more caregivers, it may have been difficult for you to become independent from your family. This may have developed into a schema based on a stunted sense of identity. This means your attempts to live by your values are met with thoughts of: 'How do I know what is important to me?' and 'Who even am I?'

Often these schemas are not known to us, so we don't notice the power they have to hijack our attempts to live a meaningful life. Studies in Schema Therapy have shown that the practice of noticing these schemas, and the thoughts that emerge from them, is an important first step to taking away their power over your life. This understanding can help us notice that thoughts are not facts. The process allows us to see that the coping strategies that we had to use when we were children to survive can be no longer helpful when we are adults. Acknowledging how these ways of thinking come from our early childhood experiences can help us find compassion for ourselves, as we are able to understand that these thoughts do not mean there is something wrong with us. They are just an outcome of our experience. I find this especially useful to help LGBTIQA+ clients understand that their schema of self-criticism and seeing themselves as less worthy can often be understood as an outcome of the stigma and lack

Goals, especially long-term ones, trick you into thinking you are completely in control of your life. But the thing is, you're not.

of acceptance they experienced when they were young. When we are treated by our families, friends and/or society as less than, this idea can become internalised as a maladaptive schema through which we interpret the world – e.g., internalised homophobia and transphobia.

It can be useful to think of automatic thoughts as a broken record player – one that just plays the same song, over and over. While the thoughts might keep returning, we can choose to notice them and remind ourselves: 'That's just my schema playing again.' And just like a record that plays on repeat, over time it gets boring. And with effort we can choose to move our attention away from these 'boring' thoughts and towards the present and living by our values. Over time we can learn how to give ourselves permission to meet our own needs – even when our thoughts tell us otherwise. Our thoughts are often stuck in the past; it is only through moving our attention to the present that we create the capacity to change how we live.

Finding the resilience to live a life of meaning in a world that does not support it

So far in this section, I have encouraged you to define your values and what a life of purpose looks like; then to examine the expectations you have of yourself, your schemas, and how you can work to move your attention away from these thoughts.

Perhaps you can see a theme here. We have spent a lot of time focused on you. What *you* want. How *you* can make it happen. But a focus on only you can be a problem. Although you may be able to define your purpose, making that life happen does not just involve you. You do not change your life in a vacuum. Attempts to change our life, towards that which is meaningful, happen within a system. And this system is generally no ally for a meaningful life.

To demonstrate this, let's take a moment to consider the difference between intrinsic and extrinsic motivation. Intrinsic motivation comes from within – the passion to complete something that is important to you. This would include learning because you are curious, exercising because it makes you feel good, or playing the piano because you enjoy it. Extrinsic motivation comes from the perception that a behaviour is going to be rewarded, or at least lead to an avoidance of punishment. This would include studying for a good grade, working to earn money, or exercising to change your appearance.

Work is not who you are, work is a place where you can enact who you are.

Examine your behaviour over the last week. How much of it was intrinsically motivated (e.g., you choose to do it because it is satisfying) versus extrinsically motivated (e.g., focused on achieving an outcome or reward)?

It is common to spend most of our time focused on extrinsic reward. And often that reward is money, people's approval, or achievement at work. This is what society has taught us is the aim of life, really - to be productive, to make money, and to purchase things so people like you.

And in many ways, this has hijacked an evolved human tendency. Our minds are focused on gathering food and items that help us survive. This tendency to gather resources was important for survival, but today it looks very different. We have become focused on buying stuff. We are obsessed with ownership. These purchases become the way we communicate who we are, demonstrate power, and meet the expectations of others. And thus, the cycle begins. We want. We work. We earn. We purchase. We want. We work ...

For many people, the pandemic has allowed us the opportunity to exit from this cycle temporarily. And in that space, we stand back, think about the cycle, and reflect if it aligns with the kind of life we want. This space allowed us to notice the disconnect that many of us experience between our behaviour and what we want our life to be. Often when we think about the life we want, we look to the future and hope our lives will turn out a certain way. We hope, but do not act. But the hard truth is that every small action you take today, and each day, adds to a week, adds to a month, adds to a year, and these years become who you are.

Our daily actions become our life and identity. So rather than focusing on long-term goals, or dreaming of the life we want, we should focus on making our daily actions be that life.

○

Taking action

When we try to change our daily actions, it often follows a pattern. We contemplate a problem, decide we need to change, set a goal, and then life happens and we just don't follow the plan. An emotional spiral can begin, sometimes starting with anger at yourself, then guilt, then shame. We start to criticise ourselves, thinking 'I am such a failure,' leading to a mindset that makes behaviour change even harder than when we started.

This is the unfortunate consequence of the individualism propagated by Western psychology. We blame ourselves when we don't achieve, because we have been taught that we can achieve anything we set our minds to. This means

that when things don't go to plan, which is inevitable
when attempting to change behaviour, we don't look
outward at all the factors beyond our control that
acted against us. We turn inward and blame ourselves.

From friends to mental health professionals to
every personal development book or religious text
you read, we are told to 'focus on what is in control
and accept what is not'. While this is important, we
need to talk about what comes next. While it is true
that a focus on factors beyond your control can be
the cause of constant anxiety and worry, it is also
true that focusing on what is in your control is not
the end of the story. I have supported many people
who are aware of what they need to do to change,
aware of what is in their control and aware of the
benefits that change would make to their lives. And
just being told to 'focus on what is in your control'
leads not to motivation, but to shame. And shame
has never helped anyone change anything.

We must find a balance between empowering
people to know they can change and helping people
find the self-compassion to know that change is
hard. And it's harder for some than others. For
example, the higher rates of mental illness, self-harm
and suicide in Aboriginal and Torres Strait Islander
communities[29] and LGBTIQA+ communities[30],
compared to the general population in Australia,
is not due to anything about the individuals
within these communities. It is due to the stigma,

discrimination, and lack of access to appropriate health care these communities face.[31]

But here is the challenge: while it is true that change in behaviour may be easier for those of privilege, it is also true that there is nothing about being a member of a minority group that means you can't take action to achieve a meaningful life. To expect less of someone based on their race, gender, abilities, or sexuality is discrimination.

This is a difficult conversation. But like all vulnerable conversations, it is the place of important change.

How do we find this balance between telling people they can make their life meaningful, at the same time as showing an understanding of the factors that act against this change? Between acknowledging someone's depression and anxiety, but also not allowing it to be a reason to not achieve the life they want. Between acknowledging the impacts of systemic racism, sexism, transphobia, and ableism, but still telling people who experience this that they should fight these systems to make a change for themselves and their communities.

I think it starts with compassion. Paul Gilbert describes a flow of compassion as having three factors: the ability to show compassion to others, to show compassion to self and to receive compassion from others.[32] I think this flow of compassion is the key to living a life of meaning.

We must aim to show compassion to others rather than telling them what they should do. This means when someone says, 'I can't,' we need to understand that saying, 'That's okay. This is hard. And I'm right here with you,' will be more likely to encourage behaviour change than saying, 'Don't worry. You got this.'

We must also teach skills in self-compassion to act against the internalised shame that so many of us face who have grown up to be told we are less worthy than others. Self-compassion is defined as the ability to challenge self-criticism through acknowledging the factors that act against you. To develop this capacity, we must build the skills through practice, and often therapy, to show ourselves kindness as we keep working towards a meaningful life.

Accepting compassion from others is perhaps the most important, because this is the moment when we can truly accept that we, like everyone else, are vulnerable. That we all struggle. And to know that this is part of what trying to live a meaningful life looks like.

Embracing uncertainty

A focus on goals creates a mindset where life is viewed as something you can control, as a series of finite goals that you can either succeed or fail at. But life is not a series of finite goals; it is one overarching process in which you have control of your actions and attitude, but little else. And, although on the surface this might not seem like a helpful idea to accept, like many uncomfortable ideas, it is one that is worth the pain. Through accepting the uncertainty, we release ourselves from the effort it takes to maintain a false sense of control. And if we can accept everything is uncertain, we can release ourselves from the rules that attempt to bring a false sense of certainty. And in that space, we can focus on the actions that are meaningful to us.

An action is not the same as a short-term goal. Actions are immediate; goals are in the future. When I ask you to think of an action that aligns with your values, I want you committing to behaviours you can do today. And yes, these daily actions may add up to the same goals you may have defined, but a focus on actions rather than long-term goals will change your experience of life. Rather than a life defined by waiting for future success, each day becomes an opportunity to live a life of purpose. Rather than your worth being determined by the success of goals (largely outside your control), your worth is determined by the intention behind your daily actions.

A focus on daily actions doesn't mean you don't achieve long-term goals; it just makes the journey there more satisfying. It will also mean that the only long-term goals you will achieve will be the ones that are meaningful to you, rather than those that are just based on society's expectations.

A focus on living by our values is also important as it allows us to have a sense of autonomy and competence in our life, no matter what our circumstance. This is because, although the way you live by your values will change, dependent on context, the intention behind your actions will remain constant, and your intention can be your measure of worth and success. While the how we live must respond to factors beyond our control, the why we live remains unbroken. As described by Viktor Frankl, 'life is never made unbearable by circumstances, but only by lack of meaning and purpose'.[33]

Now you may be thinking, this is all good and lovely but, in the end, I work for money, so the work I do is not meaningful. The other pillars of your life may provide purpose and work can be a necessary and tolerable cost. However, no matter the job or context we find ourselves in, we can always choose our attitude and actions. For example, we can notice that working in a job earns money that may be used

Values are useless if they just remain an ideal.

to care for family, so it's an action aligned with values of love and care. Or within our job we can ensure we treat people with respect, an action of kindness and connection. And the more we can live by our values at work, the more we can dismantle the divide between life and work.

On many mornings when I sat down to write this book, I felt stressed and frustrated. I became overwhelmed by the uncertainty. Will anyone like it? Will anyone find it helpful? Will anyone buy it? But then I chose my response. I chose to see those emotions as normal. And then I chose to sit down and start writing, because writing this book was an action aligned with my values of authenticity, courage, care, and community.

I can't know what will happen once the book is released. But writing it was an action of purpose I was in control of. And, through that action, I find my self-worth no matter the outcome.

PS: I do hope you like it though.

New rules in action · New rules in action

Who am I?

Imagine someone you love gives a speech about you at your 80th birthday. How do you want them to describe you? How do you want them to describe the type of person you have been with other people in your life? What words do you want them to use to describe the way you have lived? These are your values. I've written the following list to help. Remember, when choosing your values, you should be asking yourself: if I was living by this value, would it feel like I was living a life of meaning?

Write your values down (remembering they might not be included in the list on the next page) somewhere and define what the terms mean to you. I would suggest you narrow it down to five, as it can become hard to keep more than that in mind (but it's your life, so choose whatever works for you).

The New Rulebook

Acceptance	Accountability	Achievement	Adaptability
Adventure	Ambition	Authenticity	Balance
Beauty	Collaboration	Community	Compassion
Competence	Confidence	Connection	Contribution
Cooperation	Courage	Creativity	Curiosity
Dedication	Dependability	Diversity	Efficiency
Environment	Equality	Ethics	Excellence
Fairness	Faith	Flexibility	Forgiveness
Freedom	Friendship	Fun	Generosity
Grace	Gratitude	Growth	Health
Honesty	Hope	Humility	Humour
Inclusion	Independence	Initiative	Integrity
Intuition	Joy	Justice	Kindness
Knowledge	Leadership	Learning	Legacy
Love	Loyalty	Nature	Openness
Optimism	Order	Patience	Peace
Perseverance	Power	Pride	Recognition
Reliability	Resourcefulness	Respect	Responsibility
Safety	Security	Self-respect	Serenity
Spirituality	Success	Teamwork	Travel
Trust	Truth	Understanding	Vision
Vulnerability	Wealth	Wellbeing	Wisdom

Pillars of life

Write down the different domains of your life: your pillars. Aim for about four to five. Some examples might include family, friends, relationships, spirituality, festivals, music, art, work, education, sport or health.

Imagine a documentary maker had been taping your life over the last six months. Consider what you would see if you watched the tape. How have your actions aligned with your values?

Give yourself a score for how much you have lived by your values in each pillar over the last six months – with 10 meaning you have completely lived by your values, and 0 meaning your actions have not aligned with your values at all.

Your identity is made up of your actions across all parts of your life. However, it is normal for our time and energy to sometimes be focused in just one domain. Which pillar do you need to give some love to?

Think small

Pillar	Values	Actions

As discussed, values only find meaning when put into action. So choose two pillars - perhaps the ones which had the lowest scores - then, using the template provided above, write down the values from your set that are most important within these pillars. Then write down two actions that aligned with one or more of the values. When setting actions, keep in mind the following:

1. Think small - nothing big - think ridiculously achievable, and something you could do today or this week.

2. Check in: how motivated are you to achieve this? Give yourself a score out of 10. Less than 8 out of 10? Then it's likely not going to happen. Try a different action that feels more meaningful to you and more achievable.

3. Consider what thoughts you may need to notice and move your attention from.

4. Achieved it? Reward yourself.

5. Didn't achieve it? Be kind and carry on. Remind yourself that you are not the problem; the action was just unachievable. Think of another one and try again.

Two-day diary

We often feel like there isn't time to add new behaviours to our lives. However, when we examine our daily actions more closely, we can start to see how much time we may be giving to things that are not important to us. The space for meaningful actions often comes from limiting behaviour that is not meaningful.

1. Record all your behaviour for 48 hours; e.g., write what you are doing each hour.

2. At the end of the 48 hours, examine the way you have spent your time. Which actions were aligned with your values?

3. Consider which behaviour you could limit to make space for more meaningful actions.

How to make a satisficer choice

To promote a satisficer mindset (i.e. increase the likelihood of satisfaction from life), take the following steps.

1. Write down a few clear criteria for what you want from this decision; e.g., what are your most important needs?

2. Keep focus on these criteria as you look at the choices. Remind yourself that increasing the number of choices tends to decrease satisfaction.

3. Choose the first option that meets your criteria.

How to fail better

1. Acknowledge and process your emotions (see How to move through emotion on page 64).

2. Consider what was in your control and how you lived by your values through this action. What were your measures of success?

3. Take a step back and put this in perspective. What did you learn from this? How are you living by your values in other aspects of your life? How can you view this as just one moment in the long process of your life?

How to have fun

Bringing fun, joy and pleasure into your life is serious business. Here are three steps and some questions to help you along the way.

1. Know what is fun for you.

   * What brings you pleasure?

   * Who is a good person to have fun with?

   * When was the last time you felt joy? What were you doing?

2. Change your behaviour to make space for it.

   * How can I organise my life to have more fun?

   * What am I perceiving as more important than joy?

   * What is some fun I could add to today? To this week? In the future?

Love

Old rule

Love is about
finding the one.

New rule

Love is the actions
of connection,
belonging, and safety.

For nobody else, gave me a thrill
With all your faults, I love you still
It had to be you,
Wonderful you,
It had to be you.

- It Had to Be You, **Isham Edgar Jones**
  and Gus Kahn

Who doesn't want to find 'the one', right? That person who completes you, with whom there is a spark, then fireworks and then a burning love that never dies.

When you find the one, it's easy. The search is over, you've found love. You feel it. It's undeniable.

If it starts to feel like work, becomes difficult, or it just doesn't feel like it used to, this means we have not found the one. So, we should end it, and head back out to find the one, because with them it would be different.

In many ways we talk about love like it is a hole. A beautiful hole, but a hole nonetheless. A hole that we search for and then, when we find it, fall into, and we can't get out because we are in it. Deeply.

But love is not a hole. Love is not something we fall in. It is something we do.

What is love?

Often the most important question we seek to answer in life is, 'How can I love and be loved?' The idea that you will just know love when 'you feel it' is romantic but also useless. I mean, it feels good to love. But this definition limits us. Because it allows us to view relationships that aren't good for us as love. If we define love by the feeling, then anything can be love.

Until we build a common understanding of love, it remains a nice idea but not a useful concept to help get us what we need. We need to define it, because that is the only path to learning how to do it better. And we must learn to do it better.

I believe the best way to define love is to return to an understanding of our core social needs. Underneath every yearning for a romantic love or friendship, there is a biological need for connection.

Belonging is in our biology. Our bodies have evolved to know that acceptance by a group is vital for survival.[34] The prehistoric person who was outcast was not likely to have access to shelter, food, or safety. On the other hand, the person who developed and maintained strong relationships had both a survival and reproductive advantage.

Being alone is a threat to our safety, and our body reacts to let us know. There is a reason we describe the end of a relationship as heartbreak, or rejection from a group as hurtful. Our bodies experience social rejection as a physical pain.[35] We feel it.

The body is designed to connect to others through a wonderful little hormone named oxytocin. This hormone acts like a neurotransmitter, which is released to promote social bonding behaviours that are vital for survival.[36] Oxytocin is the reason kissing and cuddling feel good, why we feel more connected to someone after sex, and why parents feel such a bond to their children. However, recent research highlights that this 'love hormone' is dependent on feeling safe.[37] Our brains have not evolved to make us happy when we are touching or hugging just anyone. Oxytocin improves our mood when we are bonding with someone with whom we feel safe and connected.

This understanding of neurobiology reflects what we instinctively know to our core: humans need social connection to belong and to feel safe. What would life look like if this became our focus? Not a search for the one but taking action to become more connected in all your important relationships? Not a looking for love but taking action to make sure you feel safe? Not a hope of finding love, but behaving to belong.

That is what love is. A commitment to the actions that promote connection, belonging, and safety for ourselves and our relationships. Love is an action, not a noun.

Love is an action, not a noun.

The rules of love

According to the books and films I grew up with,
I was meant to meet a girl, fall in love, and get
married. These were the rules and, if I followed them,
I was promised happily ever after. But that's not quite
how life turned out.

When it comes to love, I'm a bit of a rule breaker.

To begin with, I fell in love with boys. Lots of
them. And for most of my life, that meant I couldn't
get married. This meant my early attempts at
belonging, connection, and safety, like those of so
many of my LGBTIQA+ friends and community,
were challenged by experiences of homophobia,
hiding who I was for my own protection, and the
knowledge that people believed there was something
wrong with me.

Yet through the pain of being excluded from
the relationship norms, I have been given the
opportunity to consider what a good relationship
looks like for me; to examine which parts of the
relationship models that surround me I want, and
which I don't. For example, I'm engaged but I also
have another boyfriend (see, told you I was a rule
breaker). I have been in monogamous relationships,
but later found that consensual non-monogamous
relationships worked better for me.

This is what being queer has come to mean to me.
I couldn't play by the rules, so I got to write my own.

This is what I want for you too. Not to be queer (unless that is who you are!), but to give you the space to step back from the expectations and rules about how relationships must be, to determine what works for you. This is not about telling you what your relationships should look like; this is about questioning all the structures that are already doing that.

○

What's love got to do with it?

Let's for a moment remove the labels we have created to define human connection. Imagine there is no dating, fiancée/fiancé, marriage, husband, wife, friend, lover, primary partner, or best mate. Imagine there are just people needing to belong, connect, and feel safe. What would be the best way to give these people what they need?

As we have already established, the rule to find 'the one' may not be working for you because your body and brain have evolved to know that belonging and connection to a group is safer than connection to one person. One person can't meet your need for belonging. Our bodies don't need to be married; they need social connection. Yet societal expectation encourages, if not demands, that your relationship with your one true love be held above all others. Is this the best way to encourage belonging?

Why are certain kinds of relationships held as more important than others? Why is the person you marry viewed as more important than someone you have been close friends with for decades? Or why should someone you are having a monogamous relationship with be prioritised above your family or friends?

With this perspective, it is also useful to consider another rule that many of my clients are starting to question or have already decided does not work for them: monogamy.

In a time before contraception, monogamy was all about ensuring men could maintain a sense of control over reproduction and therefore their estate and wealth.[38] Luckily times have changed, but the expectation for monogamy has not. Somewhere along the way, monogamy became subsumed by the romantics. And let's consider what impact this has on our relationships. Through the rule of monogamy, love and commitment are expressed through restraint rather than action. To be faithful does not require showing love, you just must not have sex with anyone else. Love became more about what you weren't allowed to do, rather than what you should be doing to show commitment.

I am not suggesting that monogamy is the root of our problems here, but it may be helpful to think of it as a choice, rather than a rule. And for many people it is a choice that will work for them and their relationship. But for others, stepping away from this socially constructed ideal may allow a freedom from the reliance on just one person to provide all needs – not to mention taking the pressure off your person to provide all the care, emotional connection, sexual intimacy, financial support and parenting support you need.

Speaking of parenting, this is the other expectation that you may be experiencing: that it is up to the biological parents to provide care for a child. Numerous studies show that there is nothing about a two-person, male-and-female partnership that is most helpful for a child's development.[39] The best environment for a child is one where their physical and emotional needs are met by responsive caregivers. The gender of that caregiver does not matter. The number of caregivers does not matter. The only thing that matters is the degree to which a child's needs are met.

It takes a village to raise a child, and two people are not a village.

One person can't meet your need for belonging. Our bodies don't need to be married; they need social connection.

Who to love?

If I am suggesting that we should move away from a focus on connection to just one person you may be wondering, how many people should we love?

Evolutionary psychologist Robin Dunbar has a theory that has stood the test of time.[40] Based on research comparing the size of the part of our brain that deals with language and emotions to the total size of our brain, Dunbar proposed that human brains can only handle around 150 stable relationships at once. And after a couple of decades studying this, Dunbar outlined what these 150 relationships look like. Through collecting data from thousands, Dunbar found that we cognitively tend to structure our social networks in specific layers of graduated closeness.

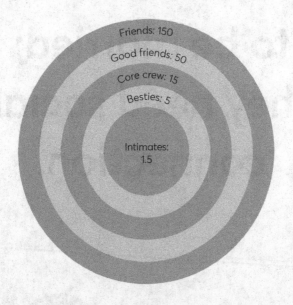

Friends: 150
Good friends: 50
Core crew: 15
Besties: 5
Intimates: 1.5

The layer you are most close to, the 'intimates', is made up of 1.5 people (an average of 1-2). Then there are 5 people, the 'besties' - the ride-or-die friends who you would drop everything to support. Next, we have about 10 friends who complete the most meaningful group of 15, let's call them your 'core crew'. Dunbar defines this as the group with whom you share your fun times, your main social connections, and the people you would trust to look after your children. The next layer of 35 (to make 50) are your 'good friends', who you'd invite to a barbecue, and the next 100 complete the 150: your wedding-and-funeral group of 'friends'. Although the number in each layer may differ slightly between individuals (e.g., extroverts tend to have more people per layer than introverts), Dunbar has shown this average structure holds up from military fighting units to Facebook groups.[41]

Dunbar presents that it's important to consider these layers, as our time for social interaction is not infinite. We need to consider how to spend our time, knowing that the strength of our relationships is dependent on the actions we take with the people in our lives. Importantly, these layers are not defined by family bonds or history, but by action.

There is a hierarchy appearing here that is useful to notice. And perhaps this shows why labels for different social relationships have come to be - e.g., close friends versus best friends versus party friends.

Dunbar's research suggests there is a biological drive to connect to a few people, in a deeper, stronger way. But rather than defining this hierarchy based on marriage, gender, patriarchy, or just because you went to high school with someone, we can base it on something else: the degree to which you are committed to taking action to promote connection, belonging, and safety.

So rather than focusing on commitment to one person through the structures of monogamy and marriage, we can focus on commitment to our most meaningful and important relationships. According to Dunbar, you have the cognitive capacity for about 15 of these relationships.

To put it another way, at any one time you have the capacity to have 15 people in your life whom you can love. Some may be your family. Some may be your partners. Some you may have sex with. Some you may marry. Some may help you raise children. They will change throughout your life as you will end those relationships with people who cannot act with love. But all will be people you love. Your kinship. Your logical family. Your community.

And this love is not just a feeling, it is shown through a willingness to take the actions of connection, belonging, and safety for these special few. So we had better be clear about what these actions are.

Connection

I started my career as a child psychologist. However, I learned quickly that this meant I was a parent psychologist. And while I was prepared to help parents in supporting their children, I was not expecting how much this would be about the parents' relationship with each other.

To help, I turned to further study and trained in emotion-focused therapy (EFT). Based on the neuroscience of love, EFT aims to provide a safe space for people to challenge cycles of conflict through emotional experiences.[42]

Through this training, my work with couples over the past decade, and my own relationships, one of the most important ideas I've learned is this: it is not conflict that is the enemy of relationships, but emotional distance. And the path back to connection is through conversations grounded in vulnerability and emotion.

The neuroscience of love shows us that our bodies are hard-wired to focus on the threat of disconnection. This may be especially true if your caregiver/s were inconsistent in responding to your needs as a child, through which you may have developed an 'anxious attachment style'.[43] This may mean that in certain relationships you become triggered to fear abandonment, need constant reassurance, feel intense jealousy, and become focused on meeting your partner's needs rather than expressing your own. However, anxious attachment (like all attachment styles – see *Polysecure*[44] for a great summary) lies on a spectrum across all our relationships, meaning that we may all from time to time make meaning from even the smallest change in the tone of voice or facial expression from a friend, or analyse every text message from a partner, looking for evidence not of love, but of risk. In the space waiting for messages after a date, our brain predicts the worst, not the best.

We feel all this fear, but then we don't talk about it.

And this leads to a devastating relationship dynamic that underlies so much dysfunction: we avoid difficult conversations and conflict, because we see those conversations as a risk to our relationship, when in fact those conversations are often the only thing that will save it. We focus on the avoidance of emotional vulnerability at the cost of our relationships.

Connection therefore needs to be based on actions of emotional vulnerability to oppose this avoidance so often experienced in relationships. These are skills in having difficult conversations, coming together after conflict, and sharing emotions with each other. This comes not only from vulnerable conversations, but also in taking action to attune to your partner's emotions and to create a space where they feel they will be accepted and understood.

This is the type of connection that not only defines love but saves it.

Belonging

Belonging is not a concept we often discuss in reference to relationships with a partner, or family relationships. We can belong to a group, but we can't belong to a partner. Yet belonging is such a useful component of love, as it highlights the fact that love demands not only authenticity, but also the self-confidence to express that authenticity. It helps us understand that the foundation of love must be self-acceptance.

As defined by Brené Brown, 'we can feel belonging only if we have the courage to share our most authentic selves with people, our sense of belonging can never be greater than our level of self-acceptance'.[45]

Beyond expressing authenticity, we also promote belonging in our relationships through intentional gathering. So often in life we may bring people together based on tradition that no longer serves the people gathered, rather than with thoughtful purpose. As described by Priya Parker in *The Art of Gathering*, we need to make purpose our bouncer.[46] We must take the time to define the specific and unique purpose of each gathering and how best to put that purpose into action. Without a thoughtful purpose, we may miss the opportunity to make people feel like they belong and, therefore, are loved.

We need to spend less time searching for 'the one' and more time building a sense of belonging and connection to the people who are already in our lives.

Safety

If someone acts to cause or threaten harm, this
is not love.

This is the advantage and the challenging
truth that comes from defining love as an action
rather than a feeling. Love becomes measured by
action. A person cannot harm you and love you
simultaneously. However, if you grew up in a family
where you were verbally or physically abused or
emotionally neglected, you may have been taught
that this was love. bell hooks, writing in *All About
Love*, has helped me understand this idea further:
'Love and abuse cannot coexist ... Too many of us
need to cling to a notion of love that either makes
abuse acceptable or at least makes it seem that
whatever happened was not that bad.'[47]

This is how a definition of love as action both
helps and hinders. Although the definition may
cause pain in the acceptance that our relationships
were, or are, not loving, it also offers a path towards
knowing what a loving relationship should be. To
know we deserve love must also mean we are able
to name how that love must be shown. We need to
know what the actions of love are, so we can love
and be loved.

Your nervous system is constantly, beyond your
consciousness, monitoring the environment to
decide if you are safe.[48] That's why you may react

irrationally and intensely in a relationship - your nervous system reacts to protect you before you even start thinking about it. And once our threat response initiates, we focus on the need to protect rather than connect. We attack or give the silent treatment. And in response, our partner reacts to this threat. A cycle begins that leaves both partners feeling unsafe, but also not willing to change.

We remain stuck, because we need to feel safe before we will make ourselves vulnerable, but we need to be vulnerable to make our partner/s feel safe. However, as Esther Perel teaches us, 'It takes two people to create a pattern, but only one to change it.'[49]

So how can we promote emotional safety for ourselves and our relationships? Sometimes safety will come through ending a relationship. However, if we are willing to work at a relationship, on an individual level, we can start by helping our nervous system to feel safe. We can act every day to promote calm regulation of the nervous system (see page 69 for strategies). We can increase our sense of safety through actions of predictability, routine, and stability.

In relationships, safety also comes from clear communication and trust. And this trust must not just be based on structures (e.g., 'I'm your partner, you should trust me'), but earned through actions that show accountability, integrity, and reliability. For example, in intimate relationships this would include clear communication to establish the boundaries of sexual or emotional intimacy with other partners, and both partners being accountable to these boundaries. Safe is sexy, because safety is the foundation that allows relationships to be fun, spontaneous, and creative.

We can also promote a sense of safety in our relationships through learning how to have a difficult conversation, apologise, and come together after conflict (see strategies on pages 141-143). Through practice, conflict and difficult conversations can become no longer perceived as threats to be avoided or fights to be won, but rather as opportunities to learn what your partner/s need and a path to strengthen your relationships.

○

Love is all you need

Most of us know what it means to tell someone 'I love you,' or to know that we are 'in love' with someone. It feels like a big deal because it is. But to be in love with someone should not be viewed as a commitment to the person – but rather a commitment to the actions of love. Rather than defining love as grounded in the false certainty provided by the structures of engagement, marriage, the promise of being best friends, or monogamy, love is achieved through the actions of connection, belonging, and safety.

When we start defining relationships by how much effort we are willing to put in, everything changes, as now the ticket to belonging is not to find your soulmate, but rather to commit to making all your important relationships work. Of course, these relationships may be with people you marry, but also with partner/s, friends, and family. All of these relationships are equal in their capacity for you to love and be loved.

And yes, I am defining them as love relationships. Because I am talking about the kind of friends you love. The colleagues you love. The family you love. I understand this may be challenging, but just like we do with family, I am suggesting we remove the idea of love from sex. Although sex may be an action of love in some of your relationships, sex is not a measure of love.

We must challenge the structures that define married and intimate relationships as paramount. These false hierarchies that mean someone who is 'single' is viewed as someone who is lacking. Those who are lacking are not those who aren't married or are not in 'a relationship', but rather those who are not in relationships in which they experience connection, belonging, and safety.

Love should not be defined by a promise, symbol, or structure; it should be deeply felt and experienced through the actions of love.

Love should not be defined by a promise, symbol, or structure. It should be deeply felt and experienced through the actions of love, for actions speak louder than not only words, but also vows.

This is the shift we need. We need to spend less time searching for 'the one' and more time building a sense of belonging and connection to the people who are already in our lives. We need to spend less time planning our wedding, and more time planning how we will commit to the actions of love. We need to shift from dreaming of how much better it would be in a new relationship, to taking action to improve the ones you already have.

The pandemic led to dramatic changes in our relationships. We experienced relationship break-ups, lost contact with friends or, most significant of all, lost loved ones to COVID-19. Our workplaces, which for many were a place of belonging and connection, now look very different. As we attempt to find our way back to each, we need a road map.

Many of us are lonely and have a yearning for social connection. But it won't just happen. It requires intentional action. It requires love.

Perhaps this is what this time of shifting sands in response to the pandemic can provide us: an opportunity to construct our lives to focus on the type of social connection that we need, not the ones we see on screens. To focus not on finding love, but on taking action to show up for our existing relationships. Not on searching for 'the one', but on constructing your life to support connection, belonging, and safety.

New rules in action • New rules in action •

Actions of connection

Check in

Set up a regular time so people can share how they feel
the relationship is going, show gratefulness for actions of
love, and discuss what they need to experience connection,
belonging, and safety.

Be vulnerable

Share not just the surface emotions (e.g., anger or stress), but
the emotions often happening underneath (fear or hurt). This
might require grounding exercises to help you stay present
and open (see page 69), and having conversations in contexts
where you feel most safe.

Maintain physical connection

In some relationships this may look like hugs, kisses, massages, or simply holding hands. In others, sex may be an important way to experience and express connection. But just like love, good sex doesn't just happen, especially in long-term relationships. It's maintained through work focused on communication, consent, learning what brings you and your partner/s pleasure, and challenging unhelpful beliefs that we often learn about what our sex should be like.[50] Everyone deserves pleasurable sex, but the path to great sex is often an individual journey. Sex therapists will be excellent support on this journey, so reach out early (the QR code on page 10 will be a good place to begin).

How to listen

Turn toward: It is common for us to become distracted by thoughts, emotions, or phones during conversations. Try to notice when you become distracted, and consciously choose to return to listening. It can be helpful to ask yourself, 'What is their experience of this?', 'How are they feeling right now?', or 'What am I doing to show that I am listening?'

Don't speak: If you are speaking, you are not listening. Avoid interrupting. Remind yourself that you will have your turn.

Validate emotions: Ensure that, when emotions are shared, you show an acceptance and empathy through statements such as, 'That sounds like a really hard place to be; I'm right here with you,' or, 'It's normal to feel hurt right now.' Avoid statements that try to make the person feel better but do not validate their emotions, such as, 'Don't worry, you'll get over it,' or, 'Just stay positive – you've got this.'

Reflect: Check in that you have understood what has been said through paraphrasing. Importantly this should be said tentatively, with a sense that you are open to being corrected. For example, 'Let me check I've understood you correctly ...' or 'So, from what I'm hearing ...'

How to apologise

It's important to examine what stops us from making a clear apology. We often get stuck as we will not take responsibility for our part until the other person accepts their part too. But that is not what apologies are about. An apology is one way. It should not be dependent on the actions of the other person.

1. Take accountability. Name your part.
2. Say, 'I am sorry.' The actual words.
3. Describe how you will change your behaviour to ensure it doesn't happen again.

How to have a difficult conversation

Focus on the why: Notice your brain's bias to focus on the reasons not to have the conversation and choose instead to focus on the long-term benefits of this conversation. Why is it important for you to have this conversation? Try to keep focus on this intention.

Be open to emotion: During the conversation, check in with your body and how you are feeling. Remind yourself that these emotions are not a threat, they are a normal part of having difficult but meaningful conversations.

Speak from your perspective: Focus on expressing your experience of events and how those experiences made you feel; e.g., 'My experience of this was ... and I felt ...'

How to come together after conflict

Consider how safe you feel to have this conversation. If you do not feel safe, reach out for support (see the QR code on page 10 for more information on phone lines and support services).

1. Try to come together as soon as possible after the conflict. Although it is normal to want to avoid the conversation, try to remind yourself that until you process the conflict, you will not be able to move on from the sense of disconnection.

2. Before you begin, ask yourself the following questions:

   * Why is it important to have this conversation?
   * When is the right time to have this conversation?
   * What might signal that we should take a break from the conversation? What will I notice in my body?

3. Set up some general rules together; e.g., we can take a break if needed; when you are listening, you shouldn't speak; and avoid 'you' statements, such as, 'You never listen.'

4. Start with vulnerability. Useful ways to do this are by expressing how the conflict made you feel or by taking responsibility for your part.

5. Commit to action: both commit to what you will do to prevent conflicts like this happening again (e.g., self-care or avoiding certain behaviours). Make a time in the future to check in on how this is going.

6. Ending it right: consider the following questions when deciding to end the conversation:

* Do we both feel completely understood?

* Is there anything else we need to discuss before we both feel we can move on from this?

* Are we both feeling ready to end this conversation?

Actions of belonging

Be authentic

Ensure you are saying what's on your mind and living by your values. Notice the expectations and rules that tell you to behave in a certain way and choose to be yourself.

Express the love

Through whatever means, tell people what they mean to you and what you love about them. And not just on birthdays - aim for every month. For example, a surprise note on the bathroom mirror, a card sent to their workplace, or an unexpected phone call.

Gather intentionally

Bring people together with purpose. Whether it be a date, dinner, or party, consider the purpose first, and then organise based on that purpose. Ideas might include celebration of achievements, relationship milestones, shared spiritual or cultural celebrations, or rituals that become defined by the relationship (e.g., monthly date nights).

Actions of safety

Communicating boundaries

Boundaries are limits we set in relationships based on our own needs. They communicate to others what our expectations are and when they have been crossed. Boundaries can help us feel safer in our relationships as they make the behaviour of others more predictable.

It is important to state that while boundaries can promote emotional safety in your relationships, if you believe your physical safety is at risk, know that support is available (there are phone numbers of services available 24/7 – see the QR code on page 10).

Boundaries must be communicated. When doing this, it may be helpful to acknowledge the impact this boundary may have but not take responsibility for another person's emotions; explain why this boundary is important to you and name the consequences of crossing the boundary. Below are some examples of what communicating boundaries might sound like in your relationships:

With partners

'I know this might be difficult to hear, but I need to be alone for the next hour.'

'I am feeling overwhelmed right now. Can we take a break and come back in 20 minutes?'

'I know we can have sex outside the relationship, but it feels like you are dating other people. Can we talk about the boundaries for our relationships with other people?'

With family

'I respect your beliefs, but if you continue to say things that are not respectful to my friends, I will have to leave.'

'I know you want to show our kids how much you love them, but please ask them if they want a hug and respect them if they say no.'

'I know this is taking time for you to understand, but it is important to me that you use my correct pronouns.'

With friends

'Although I have been able to help you in the past with things like this, I can't help you today.'

'I would love to come to your birthday, but I can only stay until 9 pm.'

'I know you meant it as a compliment, but it would help me if you did not make comments about my body.'

With workmates

'I know this is important to you, but I do not have the capacity to help you right now.'

'I do not respond to emails outside of work hours, but I'm happy to continue this tomorrow.'

'I'd like to hear what you have to say, but we need to hear from the person who was speaking first.'

Body

Old rule

Be body positive.

New rule

Develop a relationship
with body focused on
function, pleasure,
and rest.

I blame Descartes.
'I think; therefore I am.'
It's an idea psychology has taken and run with.

So much of our theories and the way we have understood mental health has been focused on the cognitive – on how we think. How we can challenge our thoughts to change our mood. How we can modify our thoughts to cure our anxiety. That changing thoughts is the key to changing how we feel.

This was certainly how I viewed my role early in my career – that it was my job to help people think differently and that would help them feel better.

Although examining, understanding, and challenging thoughts is helpful, I think it leads to a way of looking at wellbeing that almost ignores the body. Or, at least, it views the body as just an outcome of your thinking – a one-way street. The mind influences the body, yet the body does not influence the mind – a focus on mind over matter. Yet through years of supporting people and their wellbeing, I have come to understand that we need to start with the body.

I think the promise of psychologists and 'talk therapy' is that you come and sit down and talk, and the talking makes you feel better. This perhaps creates an unhelpful story: that we can talk or think our way out of emotions, whereas often the opposite can be true. If we haven't first learned the strategies to regulate our stress response, talking about experiences can trigger traumatic responses and cause adverse consequences for wellbeing. Without a focus on and understanding of how to regulate our body, talking about difficult issues can be harmful, not helpful.

Body practitioners from embodiment and somatic practices have taught me that we must centre the body in our work. We need to understand that, rather than viewing the body as impacting the mind, or the mind impacting the body, we should view it all as one system. We need to challenge the semantic division of physical and mental health: it's just health.

Through this lens, anxiety and depression are not viewed as problems that exist within the mind (indeed, the hypothesis that depression is caused by a chemical imbalance in the brain is not well supported by evidence[51]), but rather as responses of the body to our experiences and environment. And if emotions and traumatic responses are understood as existing as responses in the body, it therefore follows that we should focus on actions of the body to manage our mental health.

We don't talk our way out of emotions; we move through them. We breathe through anxiety, exercise to process stress, scream through pain, and cry through sadness.

It is also important to observe how much focus is given to therapy and medication in the treatment of mental illness, rather than strategies based in the body – e.g., physical exercise and sleep. This is the case even though exercise and rest have been shown time and time again as the most important thing we can do for our wellbeing. An overwhelming number of studies show that, from moderate mental health challenges through to acute psychiatric illness, people feel improvement in mood not only directly after exercise, but also in the long term. In fact, regular exercise has been found to be equally effective as antidepressant medication in the treatment of mild to moderate depression and anxiety.[52]

But you know all this. Our bodies know this. So, I think the more important point is not why exercise and rest are good for our wellbeing, but rather, why we don't give them more focus in our lives.

We don't talk our way out of emotions; we move through them.

Sitting still

Imagine, for a moment, what your life would look like if it was designed around what your body needs. If you were attuned to your body and felt able to take action that aligned with your needs, what would you do differently? Would you rest more? Move more? Spend less time sitting down?

For those of us able to stand, it is useful to consider why we sit so much and what impact it is having on our wellbeing.

To answer this, let's consider a time in our lives when we were less focused on societal expectations: when we were children. Think about a kids' playground. Kids move. They play. For many, the classroom is where we first experience rules being applied to our bodies. Rules based not on what our body needs, but on what is economical. Children learn not to eat when they are hungry, but rather according to when the bell rings. Children are required to passively learn. And if they can't sit still, they get into trouble. We learn to listen to the teacher, not to our bodies.

Life becomes focused on work and productivity. As children, we must work between certain hours, go to school no matter how tired we are and, when we get home, there is homework. School is when we start to separate our lives into work and play, and this divide continues into our adult lives. For many of us, work becomes a place of stationary productivity, often staring at a computer screen.

And our body communicates to us that this is not how we are meant to live. Our eyes get tired and dry. We get back pain, wrist injuries, and wrecked necks, made worse by the makeshift 'offices' we set up to work from home. And rather than respond to our body, make changes, we learn to disconnect from our body in order to work. Rather than living in a way that works for our body, we live to work.

It is important to examine the impact this stationary productivity may be having on our wellbeing in the long term. Not only are we disconnecting from our bodies, but we may start to view our body's needs as less important than what we are expected to achieve – that our need for rest must be considered in relationship to our need to work. We sleep around work, not work around sleep. But efficiency at the cost of health is not efficiency. There is a cost. We just see this cost to our health as normal, rather than as an indicator that what we are doing needs to change.

Mirror, mirror

There is another relationship with our body that starts when we are young, and then continues to be taught through every movie, Instagram feed and TikTok.

We learn that certain bodies are better than others. And that you should do all you can to get the body that will be desired and valued by society.

Consider when this first started for you. Do you recall your parents or caregivers commenting on your appearance? Do you remember how you and your friends talked about bodies at school? When did you first look in the mirror and begin to look at your body with judgement, or compare your body to another?

For many of us, the certain type of body that is privileged in our culture is one that is thin, white, and abled. The impact this has on our relationship with our bodies and our wellbeing is significant, as the creation of a body 'ideal' leads to a relationship with our bodies based on comparison and appearance, rather than an understanding of what our body needs. Rather than focusing on what we need for our health, we focus on viewing our bodies as something we should change to gain power, relationships, and success.

While the media and its portrayal of a certain body type as beautiful and sexy has a significant influence on the way we view our own body, there is another influence that is also damaging but often goes by unchallenged: the idea that a fat body is unhealthy or, more specifically, that body weight is the same as body health. And when it comes to culprits propagating this idea, it is not just the media that is to blame. The idea that body weight is a measure of health extends across medicine, government and policy.

For example, let's take the body mass index, or BMI. This formula has remained largely unchanged since it was first developed in 1832 as a population measure, to categorise health status based on your weight and height – e.g., as underweight, normal, overweight, or obese. Although the BMI may be a quick and easy way of categorising people, it is unhelpful and often harmful to use the BMI alone when examining a person's health. The BMI does not give a full picture of a person's health; it is just a measure of body size and weight. The BMI does not consider whether weight is coming from fat or muscle, or how the fat is distributed – both key indicators in measuring health risk. If you just look at BMI and not muscle mass, a professional sportsperson may be classified as 'obese' or a thin person may be viewed as healthy, despite having other physical health issues that need to be treated.

This contributes to a type of stigma often not recognised. We see it in the school yard in the harmful words of bullies and the way people are judged on dating apps. We see it in doctors' offices when GPs infer all health problems are due to body weight, despite having no information about health behaviours. It is present when patients are told to lose weight without any other health factors being considered. This is weight stigma: the discriminatory beliefs and actions made towards individuals due to their weight and size. Although often not recognised, weight stigma is one of the most common forms of discrimination in society and has risen during the pandemic.[53] It's everywhere and, like all forms of discrimination, it is harmful for both emotional and physical health.

The instigators of weight stigma are emboldened in their discrimination by the false belief that it is motivating and helpful, because it will encourage people to lose weight and be 'healthier'. But the evidence shows a very different truth.

Studies show that far from helping people, weight stigma is more harmful to health than having a high BMI[54] and leads people to be more likely to engage in disordered eating and avoidance of exercise[55]. It also increases the risk of depression, anxiety, and suicidality, particularly when people internalise stigmatising attitudes.[56] This is why it is so important to challenge judgements based on weight and size. People claim these judgements are based on making people healthier, but they do just the opposite because, when you scratch the surface of these judgements, they are not based in helping people to be healthier. They are based in sociocultural ideas that connect thinness to hard work and health, and 'fat' bodies to a lack of willpower and discipline. They are grounded in the idea that if you have a fat body, it's your fault, and that you should work hard to lose it. And to make matters worse, because weight stigma is justified as helping people, it can come from the people you would normally go to for support.

While a certain body weight and shape is viewed as more desirable or healthier, not only do we stigmatise against those who do not have this shape, we compare ourselves against this ideal body image and view it as our fault if we have not achieved it. Weight stigma does not only entrap the stigmatised but entraps us all within the expectation to achieve the ideal.

○

Not so body positive

Within a culture focused on body appearance, eating and exercise become behaviours that are only viewed in relation to body shape and weight. Food becomes moralised as bad, 'junk', or 'fuel' rather than a source of nourishment, celebration, and connection. Exercise becomes a tactic to achieve weight loss or muscle gain, rather than an action of pleasure.

An alternative has been put forward by the body positivity movement: to radically believe that all bodies are beautiful, and that we should all love our body every day.

For some people, the practice of body love and body confidence is a powerful practice. And if it works for you, you should keep it up. However, the expectation to always love your body may not fit with your reality. Perhaps there are parts of your body that on some days frustrate you. Body positivity would be asking you to ignore these feelings, to deny your reality. For many people who have long-held negative beliefs about their body, the jump to body love may seem unreasonable and unrealistic. And the inability to meet this expectation of love may just lead to unhelpful cycles of self-blame and guilt.

Many have also argued that although the idea of body positivity is useful, the movement has left many people behind. While the body positivity movement has an ideology of loving all bodies, it has become an industry that has mostly focused on loving white, cisgendered bodies. This has left many people of colour, trans and gender-diverse people, and people with disability to feel excluded from the very movement many in these communities fought to start. Further, the movement is still focused on appearance – i.e., it is not just 'love your body', it is 'love your body no matter your weight and shape'.

I have also seen the challenges of a rule to love your body in my work supporting the trans and gender-diverse community. For some trans and gender-diverse people, their journey of transition does not include a desire to change their body, and thus a focus on body positivity may be helpful. However, other people experience their body as not aligning with their gender identity.

The experience of having parts of your body that do not match who you are leads to significant distress, known as gender dysphoria. In such cases, a focus on just 'loving your body' can be harmful, as the clear evidence shows that supporting trans and gender-diverse people in their gender identity, including medical intervention to affirm their gender, leads to significant improvements in wellbeing and reduction in suicide risk.[57]

Rather than just encouraging a positive view of the body, the body positivity movement demands it. And as negative judgements of your body are an expected outcome of a society that privileges certain body types, this movement can leave little space for people to process these critical thoughts and emotions. This is the unfortunate consequence of the mix of individualism and body positivity: self-judgements about body are not able to be processed or understood, as they are seen as bad and the fault of an individual.

Any useful model for understanding body and wellbeing must challenge the focus on body appearance, as any focus on weight and shape leads to unhelpful comparison and self-criticism. However, it must also allow people to openly process negative thoughts about their body, and to understand these as momentary and normal. Finally, the model must allow space for people to decide to change their body if doing so will lead to significant improvements in wellbeing and mental health.

The following is such a model, which aims to build a long-term relationship with your body based on function, pleasure, rest, and noticing self-critical thoughts.

○

Function

In response to body positivity, a movement termed body neutrality or radical body acceptance has emerged, which invites us to focus on the function of the body and accept it for what it is. A focus on function rather than appearance asks the question 'how can I care for my body?', rather than 'how should I change it?' - to focus on what our body does and the experience of this, rather than what it looks like. Body coach Anne Poirier states, 'On one side is body hatred, and on the other is body love ... I call body neutrality a resting place from the chaos of your mind, and from the external voices of societal pressure. This is a place where you don't have to love your body, but you don't have to hate it, either.'[58]

Through this lens, exercise is not something completed to ensure change in body shape, but something that is done for the benefits of the experience in the moment, such as the dopamine hit, stress release, or the ability to engage in something meaningful. Movement becomes something you do to improve the function of your body in the present, so you can move better and engage in a more meaningful life. Such a mindset also encourages a focus on understanding our body through its current function, rather than what it 'should' be able to do, encouraging a focus on what your body does and what it needs to do better, today.

Through a focus on function, eating is no longer viewed as an action that is calculated based on the impact on body shape and weight, but an action carried out based on listening to your body and giving it what it needs. Through this idea, hunger and satisfaction are not viewed as experiences to ignore, but important signals to help us find nourishment and health.

Rest

When the challenges we face are unprecedented, our need for rest must also be unprecedented. Perhaps the 'Great Resignation' is the only way we have been able to get the great rest we all need. In a culture focused on productivity and work, it can feel like tuning into your body's need for rest becomes a threat to be avoided. We are taught that rest is not productive, but it is.

It's important here to define the difference between rest and sleep. Rest is a broader definition and is basically when the body is not working or moving. Rest in many senses is defined by what it is not; what happens when you stop working to expectation and instead do something that aims to increase wellbeing. Sleep is a type of rest, where you become unresponsive to the environment with partial or total suspension of consciousness. It's a time when the body cycles through defined physiological stages that offer it time to restore capacity for memory, attention, and learning. So if you are feeling 'brain fog', you need to rest.

Now I'm not going to spend a lot of time here telling you why rest and sleep are two of the most important things you can do to improve your wellbeing, as I know your body has already convinced you of this with every yawn and extended blink (i.e., sleeping in meetings). I'm also aware that telling a person that they need to 'get more sleep' is often experienced as anything from frustrating to infuriating. I hate it when people tell me that I 'look tired' or 'need more rest'. If your brain is anything like mine, it immediately goes to a long list of reasons I can't rest more. However, if I stand back and examine these reasons in the harsh light of day, something becomes clear. I, like many in society, have come to see rest not as a need that must be met, but as a desire that can only be considered when I have met all other expectations.

But rest should not be a reward or afterthought. Rest should be the focus. And our body is trying to tell us this. During the day we feel tired, stressed, and sore. We find it hard to maintain attention, to think clearly, and to stay awake. My body does this, but I've learned to disconnect, to ignore these signals and push through in pursuit of some set goal or task. And it is this disconnect that I try to change, and I hope you can too.

We must learn to recognise not only what our body does to signal it needs rest, but also understand the barriers that exist in our life that stop us from giving our body the rest it needs. We need to understand that just because our body has the capacity to push through, it doesn't mean there aren't long-term impacts on our health. The steps to improve your sleep are not difficult in theory, but they are challenging in practice because they require

When the challenges we face are unprecedented, our need for rest must also be unprecedented.

going against well-worn habits of self and society.
It requires us to challenge a culture that tells us that
rest is lazy and not productive. In the words of the
founder of the Nap Ministry, Tricia Hersey, 'rest is
resistance'.[59]

Pleasure

Through a diet culture that idolises restriction of
food for weight loss, and an exercise culture that
teaches 'no pain, no gain', it is understandable that
we develop a relationship with our body that views
pleasure as a problem. A focus on diet and exercise
leads us to view our body's needs not as signals to
be understood, but as sinful, selfish desires to be
avoided. Foods that bring pleasure are viewed as
indulgent; the body's need to rest as inconvenient.

I believe a focus on pleasure is key to building a
healthy relationship with your body. I understand
what you may be thinking right now: 'But if I just do
whatever brings me pleasure, I will just eat whatever
I want and never exercise, and that couldn't possibly
be healthy!' But this mindset is an outcome of how
distrusting and disconnected we have become
from our bodies. If we truly become present to, and
accepting of, our sensory experiences, our bodies will
guide us towards actions that are healthy because

A focus on diet and exercise leads us to view our body's needs not as signals to be understood, but as sinful, selfish desires to be avoided.

that is what it has evolved to do. A focus on pleasure would not mean you stop exercising; it would mean you would find exercise that brings pleasure.

A focus on pleasure is also exactly the right perspective to have on something else we do with our body - sex. Sex therapists show us the benefits of tuning out of expectations of what sex should be and tuning in to what brings you pleasure. While we often think that great sex is something that only happens when there is great desire, it is far more helpful to work on context and communication because, while you can't just turn 'on' desire, you can do a lot to make satisfying and pleasurable sex more likely to happen. As described by Emily Nagoski (in her other brilliant book *Come as You Are: The Surprising New Science That Will Transform Your Sex Life* - trust me, just read everything Emily writes), 'The problem isn't the desire itself, it's the context. You need more sexually relevant stimuli activating the accelerator and fewer things hitting the brake.'[60]

Drinking alcohol is also something many of us do for pleasure. But it is also a behaviour many of us have a complex relationship with as we try to find the balance between hedonism and health. For those of us who drink, if we really tuned in to our body's response to alcohol, we would be forced to challenge the delicate denial of the fact many of us know to be true: it would be better for our health if we drank less.

Our body communicates this to us loud and clear with every headache and hangover. However, the body also communicates to us when our drinking brings pleasure, from the taste of celebratory champagne to the relaxation a wine may bring after a hard week. So let's listen to our body now as we ask this question:

What level of alcohol intake works for you?

Your answer here may be none. Or maybe never more than four drinks. Or, like many, you may not know yet ... or you might not be ready to answer the question. In that case, I would suggest that tuning in to your body and becoming more intentional with your drinking (see strategies on page 182) may be a great way to find out.

Tuning in to your body and doing what gives you pleasure will not lead to adverse health consequences, but rather will allow you to notice all the unhealthy actions you are taking when you are disconnected from your body. Connection to what gives our body pleasure not only leads to healthy choices but rebuilds our trust in our body. And, although it might feel wrong, doing what is pleasurable may be the first step towards understanding and validating your body and your needs.

Connection to what gives our body pleasure not only leads to healthy choices but rebuilds our trust in our body.

Noticing self-critical thoughts

I think at this point, reading this, it is fair if you are thinking something along the lines of, 'That's great, Chris, but I am still going to look in the mirror tomorrow and notice everything I don't like about my body!' That is totally normal. There is nothing you can read – indeed, nothing you can do – that will get rid of your self-critical body thoughts. And that is simply because they are there for a reason. Your brain is trying to protect you. However, unfortunately, your brain is an outcome of its environment and experience. You have been taught that being a certain weight will lead to judgement and ostracism, which is a threat to social connection, relationships, and power. As such, self-critical thoughts about your body are your brain's attempt to avoid this threat.

That's why attempts to just be 'body positive' may not be working for you. We cannot control our thoughts and, when it comes to body, we have a bias to self-critical thoughts. Yet, while we can't control them, we can change our attitude towards them. Rather than viewing these thoughts as an indicator you are doing something wrong, try to notice how they are an outcome of your experiences. This may help take away their power as you accept them for what they are. Just thoughts. And then notice your ability to move your attention to your body and listen. What function are you performing right now? What does your body need to perform this function to the best of your ability?

It's a start

As an able-bodied, cisgendered white man, I hope to contribute to a dialogue about body rather than offer clear answers. The way my body easily moves through the world and is viewed by others gives me a bias that I can notice but cannot separate myself from.

I think a core benefit of a model of health focused on function, pleasure, and rest is that it encourages a movement away from a focus on bodies other than your own. Any focus on body appearance as a measure of health will encourage comparison and self-criticism. However, a focus on function, pleasure, and rest is different, as you cannot know how functional or rested another person's body is just by looking at it. And you cannot know whether someone is doing something that brings them pleasure just by observing them. These are personal experiences and, as such, they do not encourage comparison and an ideal to live up to.

In the end, I think the intentions behind the action related to your body are more important to examine than the action itself. For example, exercise to improve the function of your body or done for pleasure will have a very different impact on your long-term wellbeing than exercise to lose weight or gain muscle, even though they both affect your physical health.

Any model that aims to improve your relationship with your body should encourage body love. However, I don't think that should be the sole focus. Rather, you should see your body for what it is and what it does. Become attuned to your body, so you can know what brings you pleasure and what doesn't. We should not encourage a society where people are spending more time trying to love their body than they are trying to create a society where no single type of body is held up as an ideal. I want you to notice your self-critical thoughts as a normal outcome of the culture – not as means for you to accept these thoughts, but as a reason to want to change the culture. In the words of Sonya Renee Taylor, activist and author of the phenomenal *The Body is Not an Apology*, 'We don't need to stop using the word fat, we need to stop the hatred that our world connects with the word fat.'[61]

However, body neutrality should also not be seen as the end to everyone's journey. For many, this may be just a step towards body love, confidence, and acceptance. And everyone should be supported to experience that loudly and proudly. In the words of Taylor: 'Concepts like self-acceptance and body neutrality are not without value. When you have spent your entire life at war with your body, these models offer a truce. But you can have more than a cease-fire. You can have radical self-love because you are already radical self-love.'[62]

Your relationship with your body should be based on noticing expectations and self-critical thoughts, and instead choosing to move your attention to how your body feels and what your body needs. And we should all take action to create a culture that allows everyone else to do the same.

Become attuned to your body, so you can know what brings you pleasure and what doesn't.

Listening to your body

Set a reminder: With so much in our lives vying for our attention, if we don't set a reminder, we go through life without taking the time to check in with our body and what we need. You may do this on your phone or choose a certain time of the day or activity where you will consciously check in - e.g., in the shower, brushing your teeth, or when you get home from work.

Tune in: Try to notice your attention moving away from your thoughts and the world around you and tune in to the physical sensations present in your body. Scan your body. What do you notice? What do you need? Movement? Rest? Food? Water? Try to notice when your thoughts move to expectations about what you 'should be doing' and move your attention back to your body, and what you need.

Plan: Ask yourself, 'Which action is most important for my health today?' and commit to making it happen. Think about what support you may need to get it done, what barriers you may face, and how you will overcome them.

How to give your body what it needs

Below are some questions to help you understand your body, what it needs, and how you can provide that. These questions may be helpful journal prompts or useful starting points for conversations with supportive people in your life. As you consider these questions, aim to maintain an attitude of curiosity, acceptance, and compassion. If some questions bring up big emotions, focus on staying grounded (see page 69 for help) and remember that emotions are all part of the process of giving yourself permission to meet your needs.

Movement

The following questions aim to move your mindset from one where the motivation to exercise comes from the promise of achieving a goal weight or body shape, toward finding movement that is pleasurable and therefore motivating in and of itself:

* Does my body need gentle movement (stretching, breathing, or walking) or something more vigorous (gym, running, long walk)?

* What type of movement do I enjoy?

* What is the most achievable version of this movement?

* What are the barriers to getting this done? How will I overcome them?

* What can I do to help maintain this movement in my life?

* How will I feel during this movement? How will I feel after?

* What will this movement help my body to do better?

Food

The following is based on the principles of intuitive eating, an approach to eating by dieticians Evelyn Tribole and Elyse Resch.[63] This is an approach that aims to develop a healthier relationship with food by getting you in tune with your body's signals for hunger, fullness, and satisfaction; it challenges the external rules and rigid thoughts that may be stopping us from listening to our bodies. This approach has been shown through research to lead to improved wellbeing, lower levels of disordered eating, reduction in body image concerns and improvements in physical health indicators (e.g., blood pressure, cholesterol levels):

* What are my hunger cues?

* Is there a rule right now that's making me tell myself not to eat something? Where did I learn that rule?

* Am I seeing some foods as bad? Why is this?

* Is indulgence possible in a healthy diet? What does that look like?

* How will I know when I am full? What will I notice in my body?

* What foods would be nourishing for me right now?

* What does it feel like to be satisfied from eating? When have I experienced that?

* Am I trying to deal with emotions through eating? Is there a more useful way to process this emotion?

Sleep

Getting adequate sleep often needs to begin with the difficult task of changing your habits and setting boundaries to create the opportunity for sleep. Some ideas for this suggested by extensive research include reducing caffeine or alcohol use, sticking to a regular bedtime, making time to relax before bed, and increasing exposure to daylight in the day while decreasing exposure to screens at night. And if you can't sleep, try to break the cycles of anxiety about not sleeping by getting out of bed and doing something relaxing until you feel tired. If you stick to these behaviours and still can't sleep, seek medical advice and the support of a mental health professional.

The following questions might also be helpful to you to create space for rest and sleep in your day:

* How will resting be productive? Will it help me relax? Recover strength? Help me think more clearly?

* How can I show myself compassion as I try to improve my sleep?

* How can I improve the quality of my sleep?

* What type of rest do I need? Deep sleep? A nap? To just close my eyes for 10 minutes?

* What are the thoughts telling me I can't rest? What are they based on?

How to use social media

Although social media can be a place that connects us to people who help us build better relationships with our bodies, it can also be a space where unhelpful beliefs about ideal body shapes and appearance can become internalised. And, as we are increasingly less able to control our news feeds, we can spend hours a day consuming images curated to keep us there, distracting us from listening to our bodies and what we need. The questions below aim to help you take a step back from your social media use and consider what it is providing you, and what impact it may be having on your life:

* Am I following accounts based on appearance only? What impact does that have on the way I view my body?

* Why do I use social media? Is there a better way to achieve that purpose?

* Can I make my feed more reflective of my values rather than what people look like? How would I do that? Why should I do that?

* Is social media impacting my ability to rest? Can I limit my use before bed? What can I do to help make that happen?

* What would life look like if I stopped using social media?

How to drink intentionally

Intentional drinking is not about convincing you to stop drinking (unless that is what you want!); it's about inviting you to define a level of drinking that works for you, keeping that intention in mind before you start drinking, and then encouraging you to use strategies to stick to that level. The questions below aim to help you change your drinking habits, so keep in mind that if you are a heavy drinker, it is important to get the support of a medical professional first before reducing your use:

* What level of drinking works for me? What can I do to help maintain that – e.g., commit to alcohol-free days, only drinking in certain contexts, or not being parts of 'shouts'?

* When was my last night out drinking alcohol that was a meaningful experience? How much did I drink?

* How can I stay more intentional with my drinking during a night out?

* Are there certain environments or contexts where I find it hard to stay intentional with drinking? How can I change this or avoid these spaces?

* What would a focus on intentional drinking give me? More time in the morning? Fewer hangovers? More money? Better health?

* What signals does my body give me when I am drinking more than I need?

Afterword

My intention for this book was to offer you new ways to care for your mental health at a time when the way we live, work, and love is changing. The world has changed. We have changed. Our ways of being in the world and finding wellbeing need to change too.

And as I write this, I know the changes are not over. I have no idea what challenges the world may be facing as you read this. And I have no idea what challenges you may be facing right now. While it makes sense to want to hold tighter to expectations and structures, hoping that following the old rules will provide stability, I am suggesting we do the opposite.

Rather than returning to rules that offer a false promise of certainty, I am suggesting we awkwardly, curiously, and compassionately move toward embracing uncertainty. And, as you find your way through this uncertainty, I hope this book offers an invitation to take up space.

Take up space to check in with your body to know how you are feeling and what you need.

Take up space to rest, even when the world is telling you to work.

Take up space with each other, to define new ways to love focused on actions of belonging, connection, and safety.

Take up space to acknowledge the systems that act against you and, when you have the capacity, take up space to try to change them.

Take up space to live every day guided by what is meaningful to you, rather than by what is expected.

In this space we can truly consider what is meaningful to us and how we can make that life happen: how we can live with purpose, because the difference between uncertainty and hope is purpose.

You don't need this book to know how to take up space; you just need to give yourself permission to do it and be willing to accept the uncomfortable emotions that must come along for the ride.

Come on. Let's get uncomfortable.

Acknowledgements

Firstly, to all my clients, you have taught me how to help and what true strength looks like.

To Nic, your love allowed me to believe I could do this. I love you (and your edits).

To Joel, your love held me as I made it happen. I love you (and your big ideas).

You have both inspired this little goodie two-shoes to see that making the world a better place often requires breaking the rules, and from that this book was born.

To Mum, Dad, Ben, and all my family, thanks for the endless support that is the foundation of everything I do. Love you. And to Harper, Larke, and Addy, Uncle Chris loves you. I promise the next book will have more pictures.

To Mark, thanks for planting the seed and the unwavering support to make this book all I wanted it to be. And thanks to you and the HarperCollins team for the edits and for making the book so beautiful.

To core cRu, and Jason, Paul, Brent, Bryony, Tim, and Zoe. Each of you were so present as I wrote this, as you have all taught me what it is to live authentically and love unconditionally. Thank you. I love you all ridiculously. (Paul and Brent, I also hope the BA energy carries through into these pages.)

To Benython, thanks for all your help navigating the nitty-gritty and for what is to come.

To Amelia, Dejan, KD, Shibby, and Largs, thanks for your wise words and conversations in the early days that really helped the book take shape.

To each of the brilliant writers and researchers I referenced in this book, thank you for your incredible work that not only inspired and informed this book, but has supported so many people to live better.

And finally, to you, the reader, for supporting this book. I am so grateful. Thank you for trusting me and my words to guide you for a little while. I hope in return you have some helpful ideas to take with you, or even pass along to the ones you love.

With love, Chris.

Endnotes

1   Tolle, E. (2005). *A New Earth: Awakening to Your Life's Purpose.* Dutton/Penguin Group.

2   Rilke, R.M. (2016). *Letters to a Young Poet.* Penguin Classics.

3   Lorde, A. (2017). *A Burst of Light: and Other Essays.* Ixia Press.

4   Cambridge University. (n.d.). *Individualism.* Cambridge Dictionary. https://dictionary.cambridge.org/dictionary/english/individualism

5   American Psychological Association. (n.d.). *Mortality salience.* APA Dictionary. https://dictionary.apa.org/mortality-salience

6   Yalom, I. (2003). *The Gift of Therapy: An Open Letter to a New Generation of Therapists and Their Patients.* Piatkus.

7   Yalom, I. (2009). *Staring at the Sun: Overcoming the Terror of Death.* John Wiley & Sons Inc.

8   Dudgeon, P., Milroy, H., & Walker, R. (2014). *Working Together: Aboriginal and Torres Strait Islander Mental Health and Wellbeing Principles and Practice.* Telethon Institute for Child Health Research/Kulunga Research Network in association with the University of Western Australia.

9   Kurzgesagt. (2017). *Optimistic nihilism.* https://kurzgesagt.org/portfolio/optimistic-nihilism

10   David, S. (2016). *Emotional Agility: Get Unstuck, Embrace Change, and Thrive in Work and Life.* Avery/Penguin Random House, 2016.

11   David, S. *Emotional Agility.*

12   Brown, B. (2021). *Atlas of the Heart.* Avery/Penguin Random House.

13   Harvard Medical School. (2020). *Understanding the stress response.* Harvard Health Publishing. www.health.harvard.edu/staying-healthy/understanding-the-stress-response

14   Nagoski, E. & Nagoski, A. (2020). *Burnout: The Secret to Unlocking the Stress Cycle.* Random House.

15   Porges, S. (2011). *The Polyvagal Theory: Neurophysiological Foundations of Emotions, Attachment, Communication, and Self-regulation.* WW Norton & Company.

16   Porges, S. *The Polyvagal Theory.*

17   David, S. *Emotional Agility.*

18   Porges, S. *The Polyvagal Theory.*

19   Leighton-Dore, S. (2021). Artist website. https://www.sadmanstudio.com/shop

20   Hayes, S., Strosahl, K., & Wilson, K. (2016). *Acceptance and Commitment Therapy: The Process and Practice of Mindful Change* (2nd edition). The Guilford Press.

21   Harris, R. (2021). *The Happiness Trap* (2nd edition). Exisle Publishing.

22   Lyubomirsky, S. (2008). *The How of Happiness: A Practical Guide to Getting the Life You Want.* Penguin Books.

23   Huta, V., & Waterman, A. (2014). Eudaimonia and its Distinction from Hedonia: Developing a classification and terminology for understanding conceptual and operational definitions. *Journal of Happiness Studies*, 15, 1425–1456. https://doi.org/10.1007/s10902-013-9485-0

24   Schwartz, B. (2004). *The Paradox of Choice: Why More is Less*. Harper Perennial.

25   Schwartz, B. *The Paradox of Choice*.

26   Huta, V., & Waterman, A. Eudaimonia and its Distinction from Hedonia.

27   Ellis, A. (1988). *How to Stubbornly Refuse to Make Yourself Miserable About Anything – Yes, Anything!* Lyle Stuart, Inc.

28   Arntz, A., & Jacob, G. (2012). *Schema Therapy in Practice: An Introductory Guide to the Schema Mode Approach*. Wiley.

29   Australian Institute of Health and Welfare. (2020). *Indigenous Health and Wellbeing*. www.aihw.gov.au/reports/australias-health/indigenous-health-and-wellbeing

30   LGBTIQ+ Health Australia. (2021). *Snapshot of Mental Health and Suicide Prevention Statistics for LGBTIQ+ People*. www.lgbtiqhealth.org.au/statistics

31   Meyer, I.H. (2003). Prejudice, Social Stress, and Mental Health in Lesbian, Gay and Bisexual Populations: Conceptual issues and research evidence. *Psychological Bulletin*, 129, 674–697. https://doi.org/10.1037/0033-2909.129.5.674

32   Gilbert, P. (2022). *Compassion Focused Therapy: Clinical Practice and Applications*. Routledge.

33   Frankl, V. (1984). *Man's Search for Meaning: An Introduction to Logotherapy*. Touchstone.

34   Baumeister, R., & Leary. M. (1995). The Need to Belong: Desire for interpersonal attachments as a fundamental human motivator. *Psychological Bulletin*, 117(3), 497–529. https://doi.org/10.1037/0033-2909.117.3.497

35   Eisenberger, N. (2012). The Pain of Social Disconnection: Examining the shared neural underpinnings of physical and social pain. *Nature Reviews Neuroscience*, 13, 421–434. https://doi.org/10.1038/nrn3231

36   Owens, A. (2021). *Tell Me All I Need to Know About Oxytocin*. Psycom. www.psycom.net/oxytocin

37   Owens, A. *Tell Me All I Need to Know About Oxytocin*.

38   Perel, E. (2007). *Mating in Captivity: Unlocking Erotic Intelligence*. HarperCollins.

39   Manning, W.D., Fettro, M.N., & Lamidi, E. (2014). Child Wellbeing in Same-Sex Parent Families: Review of research prepared for American Sociological Association amicus brief. *Population Research and Policy Review*, 33, 485–502. https://doi.org/10.1007/s11113-014-9329-6

40   Dunbar, R. (2022). *Friends: Understanding the Power of Our Most Important Relationships*. Little Brown.

41   Dunbar, R. (2022). *Friends*.

42   Johnson, S. (2011). *Hold Me Tight: Your Guide to the Most Successful Approach to Building Loving Relationships*. Little Brown.

43   Fern, J. (2020). *Polysecure: Attachment, Trauma and Consensual Nonmonogamy*. Thorntree Press.

44   Fern, J. *Polysecure*.

45   Brown, B. *Atlas of the Heart.*

46   Parker, P. (2018). *The Art of Gathering: How We Meet and Why It Matters.* Riverhead Books.

47   bell hooks. (2000). *All About Love: New Visions.* William Morrow.

48   Porges, S. *The Polyvagal Theory.*

49   Perel, E. *Mating in Captivity.*

50   Nagoski, E. (2021). *Come as You Are: The Surprising New Science That Will Transform Your Sex Life.* Simon & Schuster.

51   Moncrieff, J., Cooper, R.E., Stockmann, T. et al. (2022). The Serotonin Theory of Depression: A systematic umbrella review of the evidence. *Molecular Psychiatry,* 28, 3243–3256. https://doi.org/10.1038/s41380-022-01661-0

52   Kvam, S. et al. (2016). Exercise as a Treatment for Depression: A meta-analysis. *Journal of Affective Disorders,* 202, 67–86. https://doi.org/10.1016/j.jad.2016.03.063

53   Lessard, L.M., & Puhl, R.M. (2021). Adolescents' Exposure to and Experiences of Weight Stigma During the COVID-19 Pandemic. *Journal of Paediatric Psychology,* 46(8), 950–959. https://doi.org/10.1093/jpepsy/jsab071

54   Tomiyama, A.J., Carr, D., Granberg, E.M., Major, B., Robinson, E., Sutin, A.R., & Brewis, A. (2018). How and Why Weight Stigma Drives the Obesity 'Epidemic' and Harms Health. *BMC Med,* 16(1), 123. https://doi.org/10.1186/s12916-018-1116-5

55   Zhu, X., Smith, R.A., & Buteau, E. (2022). A Meta-analysis of Weight Stigma and Health Behaviors. *Stigma and Health,* 7(1), 1–13. https://doi.org/10.1037/sah0000352

56   Pearl, R.L., & Puhl, R.M. (2018). Weight Bias Internalization and Health: A systematic review. *Obesity Reviews,* 19, 1141–1163. https://doi.org/10.1111/obr.12701

57   Australian Professional Association of Transgender Health. (2021). AusPATH: *Public Statement on Gender Affirming Healthcare.* https://auspath.org.au/2021/06/26/auspath-public-statement-on-gender-affirming-healthcare-including-for-trans-youth/

58   Haupt, A. (2022). You don't have to love or hate your body. Here's how to adopt 'body neutrality'. *Washington Post.* www.washingtonpost.com/wellness/2022/02/25/body-neutrality-definition/

59   Hersey, T. *The Nap Ministry.* https://thenapministry.wordpress.com

60   Nagoski, E. *Come as You Are.*

61   Taylor, S.R. (2021). *The Body is Not an Apology: The Power of Radical Self-Love* (2nd edition). Berrett-Koehler.

62   Taylor, S.R. *The Body is Not an Apology.*

63   Tribole, E., & Resch, E. (2020). *Intuitive Eating: A Revolutionary Dietary Approach.* St Martin's Press.

Dr Chris Cheers is a psychologist and educator with a focus on elevating mental health in the arts and LGBTIQA+ communities. Chris is a university lecturer, an endorsed Educational and Developmental Psychologist, a member of the Australian Professional Association for Transgender Health (AusPATH) and the Australian Association of Psychologists Incorporated (AAPi), and a published academic. He recently completed a PhD at the Centre for Alcohol and Policy Research at La Trobe University. Chris is a regular contributor in the media and has appeared on the *7am Podcast*, ABC News and *Reputation Rehab* (ABC TV). His writing has been published in *Archer Magazine*, and he has featured in articles for *The Guardian*, *The Age* and *The Sydney Morning Herald*. Chris has also provided workshops and mental health consultation to arts organisations, theatre productions, universities and companies across Australia.

chrischeers.com @chrischeerspsychology

Harper *by* Design

An imprint of HarperCollins*Publishers*

HarperCollins*Publishers*
Australia • Brazil • Canada • France • Germany • Holland • India
Italy • Japan • Mexico • New Zealand • Poland • Spain • Sweden
Switzerland • United Kingdom • United States of America

HarperCollins acknowledges the Traditional Custodians of the lands upon which
we live and work, and pays respect to Elders past and present.

First published on Gadigal Country in Australia in 2023
This edition published in 2024
by HarperCollins*Publishers* Australia Pty Limited
ABN 36 009 913 517
harpercollins.com.au

A catalogue record for this book is available from the National Library of Australia.

ISBN 978 1 4607 6650 7

Publisher: Mark Campbell
Publishing Director: Brigitta Doyle
Editor: Ariana Klepac
Designer: Mietta Yans, HarperCollins Design Studio,
adapted from an original branding design by Jesse Mallon